Clinical Governance in a Changing NHS

Edited by

Myriam Lugon
Consultant
Clinical Governance and Health-Care Policy
London

Jonathan Secker-Walker
Emeritus Consultant
University College London Hospitals
London

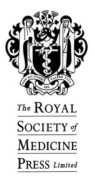

The ROYAL
SOCIETY of
MEDICINE
PRESS Limited

British Library Cataloguing in Publication Data
A catalogue record for this book is available from the British Library

ISBN 1 85315 665 5

Distribution in Europe and Rest of World:
Marston Book Services Ltd
PO Box 269
Abingdon
Oxon OX14 4YN, UK
Tel: +44 (0) 1235 465500
Fax: +44 (0) 1235 465555
E-mail: direct.order@marston.co.uk

Distribution in the USA and Canada:
Royal Society of Medicine Press Ltd
c/o BookMasters, Inc.
30 Amberwood Parkway
Ashland, Ohio 44805, USA
Tel: +1-800 247 6553/+1 800 266 5564
E-mail: order@bookmasters.com

Distribution in Australia and New Zealand:
Elsevier Australia
30–52 Smidmore Street
Marrickville NSW 2204
Australia
Tel: + 61 2 9517 8999
Fax: + 61 2 9517 2249
E-mail: service@elsevier.com.au

Typeset by Phoenix Photosetting, Chatham, Kent
Printed and bound in the UK by Bell & Bain Ltd, Glasgow

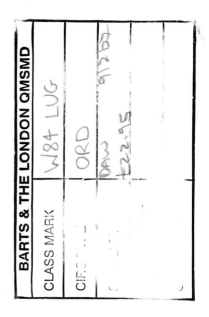

Contents

List of Contributors

Michael C Bishop
Department of Urology, Nottingham City Hospital NHS Trust, Nottingham, UK

L Peter Fielding
Clinical Professor of Surgery, York Hospital, York, Pennsylvania, USA

Steve Gallivan
Professor of Operational Research; Director, Clinical Operational Research Unit, Department of Mathematics, University College London, London, UK

Edward Griffiths
Head of Subject Division, School of Health, Community and Education Studies, University of Northumbria, UK

David Hatch
Emeritus Professor of Paediatric Anaesthesia, Institute of Child Health, London; Chairman, Performance and Health Assessment Implementation Groups, General Medical Council

Rosemary Hittinger
Group Director of Clinical Governance, HCA International, London, UK

Rowland B Hopkinson
Medical Director – Governance, Consultant in Anaesthesia and Critical Care, Deputy Chief Executive, Heart of England NHS Foundation Trust, Birmingham Heartlands Hospital, Birmingham, UK

Siân Jones
Care Pathways Manager, Service Improvement Team, Cardiff & Vale NHS Trust, Cardiff, UK

Myriam Lugon
Consultant, Clinical Governance and Health-Care Policy, London, UK

Anna Maslin
International Officer for Nursing and Midwifery, The Department of Health, London, UK

John Miller
Associate Dean, School of Health, Community and Education Studies, University of Northumbria, UK

Simon Mitchell
Regis Medical Centre PCT, Rowley Regis, UK

James Reason
Professor Emeritus, University of Manchester, Manchester, UK

Nicola Roderick
Clinical Governance Analyst, University Hospital of Wales, Cardiff & Vale NHS Trust, Cardiff, UK

Bob Sang
Director, Sang Jacobsson Ltd, Newick, East Sussex; Honorary Member of the Patients Association, Harrow, Middlesex, UK

Jonathan Secker-Walker
Emeritus Consultant, University College Hospitals, London, UK

Carol Singleton
Fellow, Faculty of Public Health, Derbyshire, UK

Louise Teare
Clinical Effectiveness Lead and DIPC, Mid-Essex Hospitals NHS Trust, Broomfield Hospital, Chelmsford, UK

Tom Treasure
Professor of Cardiothoracic Surgery, Guy's and St Thomas' Hospital, London, UK

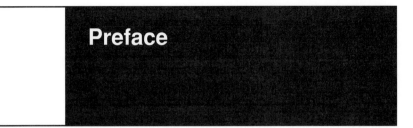

Preface

'Away with the cant of "measures not men"! – the idle supposition that it is the harness and not the horses that draw the chariot along. If the comparison must be made, if the distinction must be taken, men are everything, measures comparatively nothing.'
George Canning. Speech, House of Commons, 1801

This is the third book edited by us and published by the RSM Press relating to Clinical Governance. A number of high-profile quality failures have led to parliamentary and media demands for improved quality control of medicine. Among others, these include failures arising from paediatric cardiac surgery,[1] failures in the practice of gynaecology by some doctors, and failures related to the accuracy of breast screening. As a result the last decade has seen considerable efforts to reform the GMC, with the impending introduction of revalidation for doctors, emphasis on clinical risk management, the National Patient Safety Agency, and, of course, clinical governance – a system of quality monitoring that should cover all aspects of clinical activity.

The last decade has also seen a substantial increase in the amount of taxpayers' money invested in the NHS. In order to demonstrate to voters that the money has been well spent, numerous quangos have been set up, with varying survival rates (e.g. CHI), a plethora of targets have been launched and managers have been given the responsibility to achieve them, and a considerable degree of reliance on the independent health sector to reduce waiting lists has been introduced. Such central orchestration may profoundly affect attempts to provide regular safe high-quality care:

- Waiting-list targets may interfere with clinical priorities. Removing the treatment of straightforward diseased hips and cataracts to Independent Sector Treatment Centres (ISTCs) denies these cases for training junior surgeons and may compromise the financial viability of the local hospital. With doctors, often from abroad, rotating through the ISTCs, outcomes must be difficult to monitor and overall clinical governance difficult to implement.

- Out-of-hours primary care can also be thinly stretched – on a Saturday, one locum GP had to travel from Luton to Somerset and back in order to certify a patient dead.
- The 4-hour A&E target has had a profound effect on hospitals' bed-state.

Industry, passenger aircraft design, the armed services and supermarkets understand the necessity for spare capacity, tolerance or redundancy in order to meet the needs of safety, emergency situations and the customers of the organization most of the time. Such tolerance is seen as an essential part of good management. The NHS, however, has been praised for efficiency in having bed occupancy rates of 97% (or sometimes over 100% with 'hot bedding') and operating theatres and ICUs full to capacity all the time. Politicians, senior managers and finance officers appear to consider high occupancy rates as 'good' management, making the most of facilities and being cost-effective. The arrangement for new Private Finance Initiative hospitals usually requires a reduction in the number of acute beds, which creates problems unless a community infrastructure has been developed as an alternative to acute admission. Lack of sufficient number of acute beds produces high occupancy, which is not accounted for by 'winter pressures'[2,3] but is certain to have been adversely affected by readmissions of patients discharged too quickly in order to free up a bed and by the opting out by GPs from most out-of-hours work under the new contract agreed with the government.

The 4-hour target set by government for the maximum waiting time in A&E might seem to be a patient-friendly aspiration, but has resulted in some patients being put at risk – either by being 'admitted' within 4 hours with no ward to go to or by having to be looked after in the ambulance in the A&E yard until there is space in the A&E department. Patients on trolleys for many hours, then going to inappropriate wards and waiting for more than 24 hours for space in the emergency theatre can never be compatible with good clinical governance. The longer that elderly patients wait for their fractured hips to be fixed in theatre, the higher is their mortality. Such lack of elasticity or tolerance in the system is actually an example of 'poor' management in the service. It is seen as such by clinical staff, who recognize that a bed occupancy rate of about 85% provides the available capacity to be able to admit most patients to appropriate wards in reasonable time.

The trajectory taken by most accidents has been well described.[4] While staff at the sharp end are usually responsible for the mistake or violation that triggers an accident, the environment in which they are expected to work has an important effect on promoting the likelihood of that human error. High occupancy rates and the resultant lack of order and consistency in the admission of patients to beds in appropriate wards is a fertile environment in which the likelihood of human error increases.

High occupancy rates lead hospital bed managers to place patients in any available bed in the hope that an appropriate bed will become available in due course. These patients are usually called 'outliers'. Placing patients in inappropriate wards and then moving them to the specialist ward – maybe via other wards en route – causes profound quality problems, some of which are listed below:

- There is good evidence that clinical outcomes are better when patients are nursed by staff with specialist skills and cared for by specialist physiotherapists and other clinical staff in designated wards.[5]
- The concept of the need for care by multidisciplinary teams is lost to the outlier patient.
- Patients get 'lost' and may not be seen by medical staff for several days.
- Wards are having to attempt to care for patients under numerous consultants with different treatment requirements and regularly changing junior staff.
- Consultant rounds have to include many wards (up to 13 or more have been reported) in order to visit outliers. This takes substantial amounts of time and reduces the quantity and quality of teaching for postgraduates and medical students.
- Because of the numerous rounds by consultants and junior staff, many wards now have separate ward rounds for the nursing staff – just so that they can get on with their job. Thus, despite the need for teamwork and 'multidisciplinary care', there is often now no regular interprofessional dialogue about patients.
- The fragmented nature of junior medical staffing, especially at nights and weekends, compounds the problem of having young doctors admitting patients on up to 15 wards. The Hospital at Night scheme may help with this problem, provided there are sufficient medical staff available with the appropriate skills. When a large number of admissions occur, some patients wait hours to be assessed.
- Because of these pressures, many handovers between medical staff take place over the telephone.
- Pathology reports ordered in one ward may fail to connect with patients when they are moved to another ward.
- The care of medical patients in surgical wards denies access to specialist surgical wards by elective surgical patients. Elective surgery is thus cancelled or carried out at short notice. On-the-day admissions compromise preoperative assessment by the patient's anaesthetist.

- Discharge planning is less efficient when patients are on inappropriate wards or moved, thereby compounding the problem by increasing the length of stay.
- 'Hot bedding' may lead to less thorough cleaning of the bed area between the discharge of one patient and the arrival of the next and increase the likelihood of hospital-acquired infection, including MRSA, moving with infected patients from ward to ward.
- The information contained in the hospital patient administration system is likely to be compromised. There is confusion on the wards as to which patients have moved and to where, and who belongs to whom in terms of transfers when the PAS bed-state return is made.

The multiplicity of government initiatives and agencies attempting to modernize the health service will no doubt introduce improvements in the service to patients towards whom the cash is targeted – cardiac surgery for example. There are, indeed, more efficient ways of managing patients through the system, not least at the end of treatment, when discharge to an appropriately supportive non-acute environment is in everyone's best interest. Pathways of care can help alleviate the lack of continuity of staff providing such care and make explicit what needs to be done, and by whom, across the healthcare sectors.

New ways of working and the requirements of the Private Finance Initiative may also reduce the numbers of acute beds and operating theatres believed to be required. However, to restore some semblance of order and to improve the quality of the care that we provide to admitted inpatients, the numbers of beds and theatres must allow for a degree of tolerance and spare capacity. It is far better to have some empty beds and an immediately available theatre if we want to reduce the numerous clinical risks that a high occupancy rate brings in its wake.

While overall progress has been made in all aspects of clinical governance, the implementation across the NHS is still patchy.[6,7] This initiative has had some positive effect by integrating quality into service delivery and making clinicians and managers more accountable.[8] However, much more needs to be done to ensure that the various quality systems are better integrated and the information they generate used more effectively to be able to inform where improvement strategies need to be targeted. Clinical governance should become an integral part of everyday clinical practice, and increasingly, as networks are established, to transcend the traditional organizational boundaries.

Our first two books reviewed the mechanisms used for making clinical governance effective. This third book reflects, after five years of experience, on the problems of making clinical governance a reality – rather than a required bureaucratic pastime. This is in the light of political changes, both from the UK and the EU, which are outside the control of the organizations that must actually deliver the healthcare. Some of the following chapters reflect these difficulties and cover topics that are relevant to today's modern NHS.

References

1. Bristol Enquiry Report. Available at www.bristol-inquiry.org.uk.
2. Bagust A, Place M, Posnett JW. Dynamics of bed use in accommodating emergency admissions: stochastic simulation model. *BMJ* 1999; **319:** 155–8.
3. Morgan K, Prothero D, Frankel S. The rise in emergency admissions – crisis or artefact? Temporal analysis of health services data. *BMJ* 1999; **319:** 158–9.
4. Reason JT. The human factor in medical accidents. In: Vincent C, Ennis M, Audley RJ (eds). *Medical Accidents 1993.* Oxford: Oxford University Press, 1993.
5. Audit Commission. *United They Stand – Co-ordinating Care for Elderly Patients with Hip Fractures.* London: HMSO, 1995.
6. Commission for Health Improvement. *Emerging Themes from 175 Reviews.* March 2003.
7. Commission for Health Improvement. *What Has CHI Found in Acute Services?* March 2004.
8. Comptroller and Auditor General. *Achieving Improvements through Clinical Governance – A Progress Report on Implementation by NHS Trusts.* September 2003.

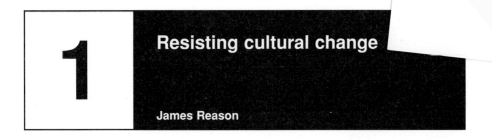

1

Resisting cultural change

James Reason

Introduction

All man-made systems resist change to some extent, not least because the status quo confers position and influence upon those in the upper reaches who play major roles in shaping the culture. And change is even harder when, like healthcare, the system in question has brought huge benefits to mankind. If it works, why meddle with it?

The answer is simple: the benefits are bought at too great a cost. Healthcare professionals – unlike aviators, for example – have never really come to terms with the inevitability of human error. This means that almost every healthcarer carries a burden of unshared guilt due to having unwittingly harmed a patient through error. The burden is made particularly onerous, not only since causing harm was the very last thing any of them wanted to do, but also because the whole ethos of medical training leads doctors and their colleagues to believe that such lengthily and expensively acquired expertise will ensure that they will get things right. But the numbers tell a different story. Several international studies show that approximately one in ten hospitalized patients (plus or minus two) are killed or injured iatrogenically.[1-5] The only thing unique about these so-called 'medical errors' is the context in which they occur: doctors, nurses and pharmacists are just like the rest of us – they are human and so make mistakes.

The notion of infallibility is deeply rooted in the healthcare culture. It leads to the belief that errors, particularly those that have bad outcomes, are manifestations of incompetence, carelessness or recklessness – for which naming, blaming and shaming are appropriate responses. This pernicious myth is perhaps the single greatest obstacle to improving patient safety. We must cease treating errors as a moral issue. Fallibility is the norm, not the exception. Errors happen in all fields of human endeavour. The trick is to recognize their inevitability. This means understanding the nature of error and the psychological and situational factors that provoke it. Errors are not random events. They take very predictable forms. The same circumstances keep on producing the same kinds of error in very different people.

It would, however, be naive to assume that we can change these entrenched views overnight. Cultural transitions take time, and in order to achieve beneficial changes, we must be prepared for the powerful psychological and organizational processes that will act against them. This chapter discusses some of the more obstinate of these countervailing forces. We begin by examining three views of human error that have constituted serious obstacles to the furtherance of patient safety.

Unhelpful perspectives on human error

Opinions on the origins, nature and management of human error vary widely. Different viewpoints lead to different models of cause, and each has its associated countermeasures. In this section, we will examine three widespread but unhelpful perspectives on error: the plague or defect model, the person model, and the legal model.

The plague or defect model

One reaction to the discovery of a high incidence of errors in healthcare institutions has been to describe them as 'a national problem of epidemic proportions'.[6] The term 'epidemic' puts error in the same league as AIDS, SARS or the Black Death (*Pasteurella pestis*). A logical step from this 'plague model' is to call for the removal of human error; but, unlike some epidemics, there is no specific treatment for error.

A closely related view is that errors are the product of built-in deficiencies in human cognition – a perspective that leads system designers to strive for ever more advanced levels of automation in order to keep fallible humans out of the loop as far as possible. These are both highly misleading representations.

The problem stems from confusing error with its occasional consequences. That errors can and do have adverse effects leads many people to assume that human error is a bad thing. But this is to ignore three important facts. First, most errors are inconsequential. Second, 'correct' performance – that is, behaviours in which the actions follow the plan and achieve their desired outcome – can also have harmful effects, as the events of 11 September 2001 tragically demonstrated. Third, errors may have highly beneficial outcomes, as in trial-and-error learning and serendipitous discovery.

There is nothing intrinsically wrong with errors. They arise from highly adaptive mental processes. Each basic error tendency is part of some essential cognitive ability. Consider the following examples:[7]

- The ability to carry out actions automatically without moment-to-moment conscious control makes us liable to absent-minded slips and lapses when our actions do not go as planned. But continuous 'present-mindedness' would make life insupportable: we would waste hours each day deciding how to fasten a button or tie a shoelace.
- The resource limitations of working memory and attention are essential for the focused execution of planned actions; but this necessarily selective ability also makes us vulnerable to information overload and the leaking of data from short-term memory.
- A long-term memory that contains specialized 'mini-theories' (schemas) rather than isolated facts allows us to make sense of the world, but it also makes us susceptible to confirmation bias – the tendency to cling on to some initial hypothesis in the face of contradictory evidence. A hunch, even a wrong one, allows us to structure our mental work. Cognition, like nature, abhors a vacuum.

Even the way in which errors are produced carries an adaptive advantage. Errors arise because the mental processes necessary for correct performance are under-specified. This can take many forms: distraction at some crucial branching point in an action programme, incomplete knowledge, sparse or ambiguous sensory data, forgetting, and the like. But, despite the many ways in which mental processes can be under-specified, the cognitive system's response is very consistent: it 'defaults' to producing actions, perceptions or thoughts that are frequent, familiar and appropriate for the immediate context. This is not necessarily logical, but it is very functional. When the human cognitive system is forced to 'guess', it produces a response that has proved useful in similar circumstances in the past.

These reactions are shaped by unconscious heuristics – intuitive rules-of-thumb – that influence how knowledge structures or schemas are selected and retrieved from memory in response to the prevailing situational demands. One such heuristic is 'match like with like' (similarity matching), and when this process identifies a number of possible candidates in long-term memory, the conflict is resolved by the 'frequency-gambling' heuristic – calling to mind (or into action) that knowledge structure that has been used most frequently in those circumstances in the past. This is why so many of our errors take the form of strong habit intrusions or 'strong but wrong' responses.

In summary: errors *per se* are not bad. Correct performance and error are two sides of the same coin. As Ernst Mach put it: 'Knowledge and error flow from the same sources, only success can tell one from the other.'[8]

The person model

The 'person' view of human error is widely held and intuitively appealing. It focuses on the unsafe acts – errors and procedural violations – of people at the sharp end of the healthcare system: nurses, physicians, surgeons, anaesthetists, pharmacists and the like. These unsafe acts are seen as having their origins in wayward psychological processes such as forgetting, inattention, poor motivation, carelessness and undesirable practice. Logically enough, the associated remedial measures are targeted primarily at the erring individuals. These countermeasures include 'fear appeal' poster campaigns, writing new protocols or adding to existing ones, sticks and carrots (mostly the former), threats of litigation, suspending, retraining, and, of course, the inevitable naming, blaming and shaming.

These reactions, as mentioned earlier, are perhaps the most potent in their harmful affects upon patient safety. Before considering these adverse consequences, however, it is worth spending a moment in understanding why these feelings are so pervasive – and so satisfying for those doing the blaming. They have their roots in a number of powerful psychological tendencies:[7]

- The *counterfactual fallacy*: in seeking causes for bad events, we are drawn to the proximal actions of those in direct contact with the patients. Our thinking goes as follows: if X had not acted as he or she did then the event would not have happened. Thus X caused the bad outcome.
- The *fundamental attribution error* is one of the main reasons why people are so ready to accept the term 'human error' as an explanation rather than something that needs explaining. When we observe someone behaving less than adequately, we explain the actions in dispositional terms. We say that he or she was careless, silly, thoughtless, irresponsible or incompetent. But if you were to ask the people in question to account for their actions, they would tell you how the circumstances had shaped their actions. The truth usually lies somewhere in between.
- The *illusion of free will* is another reason why we are so inclined to blame people rather than situations. People, especially in Western cultures, place great value in the belief that they are free agents and thus the controllers of their own destinies. Feeling ourselves to be capable of choice naturally leads us to assume that others are the same. They too are seen as autonomous, able to choose between right and wrong, and between correct and erroneous courses of action.

- Yet another factor is the *just-world hypothesis*, the belief sha⟋ children and many adults that we get what we deserve. In short, bau ᴜ.. only happen to bad people, and conversely.
- A further influence is *outcome bias* – this is the tendency to evaluate prior decision making according to whether the outcome was good or bad. The belief is that bad events can only arise as the result of bad decisions, and vice versa. But history teaches us otherwise: good decisions can still have bad outcomes.

There is some substance to the person model. People do respond to motivators, but usually only in workplaces that are personally hazardous. It is also the case that certain behaviours are indeed egregious and warrant disciplinary action; but research in other domains suggest that these culpable unsafe acts amount to less than 10% of the total number committed. And, of course, it is both managerially and legally convenient to uncouple a person's unsafe acts from any institutional responsibility. We will return to this issue in a moment.

Notwithstanding its administrative and legal convenience, the person model has two major shortcomings:

- The effective management of patient safety depends critically upon establishing a climate of trust in which people are prepared to report their errors, near-misses and 'free lessons'. But a blaming-and-shaming culture is wholly incompatible with a reporting culture. People are reluctant enough to confess their slips and mistakes without the additional threats of public disgrace and disciplinary action. Without a reporting system that collects analyses and disseminates information about patient safety incidents, a healthcare institution has no memory; and without a record of past events, it cannot learn.
- A natural consequence of blaming and shaming individuals on the frontline is to isolate their actions from the systemic context in which they occurred. Good safety information systems reveal that the same errors keep recurring in the same situations, regardless of the particular individual involved. Isolating unsafe acts from their system context prevents the institution from identifying and rectifying these error traps. All institutions have them, and the extent to which they are sought out and removed is an important indicator of the organization's safety culture.

The legal model

This is a variant of the person model, but with strong moral overtones. Central to this view is the belief that responsible and highly trained professionals should not make errors. Those errors that do occur, however, are thought to be rare but sufficient to cause adverse events. Errors with bad consequences are negligent or even reckless and deserve deterrent sanctions – echoes of the *just-world hypothesis*.

Far from being rare occurrences, the research evidence shows that highly trained professionals make frequent errors, but most are either inconsequential or detected and corrected. A recent study extrapolated the worldwide error rates on the flight decks of commercial airliners on the basis of 44 hours of continuous observation of pilot errors in flight.[9] The authors estimated that there were around 100 million errors committed in cockpits each year, but the accident records indicate that there are only 25–30 hull losses per year.

Another study[10] involving direct observations of 165 arterial switch operations (correcting the congenital transposition of the aorta and pulmonary artery in neonates) in 16 UK centres showed that, on average, there were seven events (usually arising from errors) in each procedure, of which one was major and life-threatening and the others constituted minor irritations. However, over half of the major events were identified and corrected by the surgical team. Neonatal cardiovascular surgery takes surgeons to the very edge of their cognitive and psychomotor performance envelopes. Errors are inevitable. The virtuoso surgeons make errors, but they anticipate them and mentally prepare themselves to detect and recover them. This mental and organizational preparedness – or mindfulness of danger – is one of the defining characteristics of high-reliability organizations.[11]

These and other studies make it clear that error making is the norm, even among highly accomplished professionals. Training and experience do not eradicate fallibility; they merely change the nature of the errors that are made and increase the likelihood of effective compensation. Far from being *sufficient* to cause bad outcomes, the record shows that only very occasionally are the unwitting acts of professionals *necessary* to add the final touches to a disaster-in-waiting that has been lurking on the sidelines, often for a lengthy period.[12]

The dynamics of denial

By restricting the search for causal factors to the behaviour and psychology of people on the frontline, proponents of the person and legal models create further systemic problems for themselves. Having isolated the erring individuals from the workplace in which the unsafe acts occurred, they lack any reliable information about the true nature of the local hazards, and so feel safe. While they acknowledge that there may be a few 'bad apples' in the barrel, they believe that the barrel itself – the system at large – is in good shape. Having identified and 'dealt with' the 'wrongdoers', it is but a short step to the view that it will not happen here again. And this has a corollary: the notion that anyone who says differently is a troublemaker. Blaming thus fosters denial.

The degree to which an organization disregards or denies safety-related information has been used by Ron Westrum[13] to differentiate three types of safety culture – *pathological, bureaucratic* (or *calculative*) and *generative*:

- *Pathological* organizations muzzle, malign or marginalize whistle-blowers, shirk collective safety responsibility, punish or cover up failures, and discourage new ideas. In short, they do not want to know.
- *Bureaucratic* or *calculative* organizations – the large majority – manage safety 'by the book'. They will not necessarily shoot the messenger, but new ideas often present problems. Safety management tends to be compartmentalized. Failures are isolated rather than generalized, and treated by 'local fixes' rather than by global reforms.
- *Generative* (or high-reliability) organizations encourage individuals and groups to observe, to inquire, to make their conclusions known, and, where observations concern important aspects of the system, actively bring them to the attention of higher management.

Denial of patient safety problems finds nourishment from a variety of sources. One of the most persuasive is that the epidemiological studies cited earlier do not necessarily conform to the everyday experience of individual healthcare professionals. It has been calculated that if 100 patients die each day from iatrogenic injuries in US hospitals, and there are 5000 hospitals, the rate of injury is one patient per hospital every 2 months – a virtually non-observable statistic.

Entrapment

Another process that sustains denial is what Weick and Sutcliffe[14] have called a 'culture of entrapment'. They based their analysis on the very detailed Report of the Public Inquiry into Children's Heart Surgery at the Bristol Royal Infirmary (BRI). Between 1988 and 1994, the mortality rate at this hospital for open-heart surgery in very young children was approximately double the rate of any other centre in England for most of this period. Concerns about these deaths began to surface in 1986, and continued throughout the 1990s. Parents called for an inquiry in 1996, and the formal board of inquiry was established in 1998. Its findings were published in 2001. Among its conclusions was the observation that despite the very clear evidence to the contrary, neither the senior clinicians nor their managers acknowledged that the hospital's performance in paediatric surgery was inadequate.

7

The questions addressed by Weick and Sutcliffe were how did this mindset of denial originate and why was this blindness to the facts so resistant to change. Their explanation is as follows:

> 'BRI reconstructed the history of excess deaths and transformed it into a history of excess [patient] complexity. That reconstruction rescued order from disorder and imbued the past with meaning, all of which is perfectly understandable. What is harder to accept is the persistence of the rationale that precludes learning, reduces openness to information, and minimizes cross-specialty communication. The reconstructed rationale persists because layers of bureaucrats above the surgical unit, people who had some say in the original choice to designate BRI as a center of excellence, find their own judgements in jeopardy. The unintended consequence is that the whole chain of decision makers comes to support an explanation that makes it difficult for an underperforming unit to improve or to stop altogether.'

(Reference 14: p80)

The Inquiry Report described BRI as a collection of 'tribes' – fragmented, loosely coupled, self-contained subcultures. Within each professional subculture, there is a high degree of autonomy. But this autonomy works against learning. The poor results of the paediatric surgeons were both conspicuous and irrevocable. They needed to be rationalized: 'It's a new field of surgery.' 'We're on a learning curve.' 'Our cases are unusually complex.' Weick and Sutcliffe put it very elegantly: 'Through repeated cycles of justification, people enact a sensible world that matches their beliefs, a world that is not clearly in need of change' (reference 14: p81). What begins as a plausible rationalization hardens into dogma because it makes sense of the world and reduces personal vulnerability. For these reasons, however, it also precludes learning and improvement.

Organizational silence

Most people at one time or another have found themselves in situations where they have felt unable to speak up about an issue of concern. When this reluctance to communicate problems upward is shared by many employees, it has been termed 'organizational silence'.[15]

Many of the organizational and managerial characteristics that promote organizational silence will be very familiar to many healthcare professionals, particularly to nurses and junior doctors. Here are some of them:

- Top management teams may be dominated by people with economic or financial backgrounds.
- Senior appointments to management teams may be made from outside rather than by promotion from within.
- Managerial beliefs contributing to organizational silence will be more common in stable and mature organizations.

- A climate of silence will be more likely when there is a high degree of demographic dissimilarity between top managers and lower-level employees.
- Such beliefs will be more common in organizations that rely heavily on contingent workers (e.g. agency nurses and locum physicians).
- To the extent that the top management believes (often implicitly) that employees are self-interested, and that management knows best, and where dissent is regarded as unhealthy, the organization is more likely to have a centralized, non-participatory decision making, and will be less likely to have formal upward feedback channels and more likely to reject or react negatively to input from subordinates.

When organizational silence is well established, a number of negative consequences are likely to ensue:

- A lack of critical analysis of ideas and alternatives leads to less effective organizational decision making.
- Lack of negative internal feedback leads to poor error detection and correction.
- Employees feel undervalued and powerless. These perceptions, in turn, create low trust, low commitment, low job satisfaction, greater job-related stress and higher rates of withdrawal and turnover.

Is there any remedy for this pathological culture of silence? The prognosis is not good. Creating a climate that encourages employees to speak up requires some fairly dramatic changes: a new pluralistic and empowering management team or some well-publicized adverse event that highlights the organizational penalties of silence. But, as the BRI case study showed, even institutions faced with clear evidence of less than adequate performance do not necessarily engage in global reforms. The dynamics that create and maintain silence will be hard to change, partly because they are largely unspoken and not available to direct observation, and partly because a loss of employee trust is not easily reversed. Suspicion, cynicism and fear are difficult to eradicate, particularly in hospitals where different rules seem to apply to the various professional layers of the system. Nurses, for example, can often expect to receive severe sanctions for behaviours that may be excused or explained away in senior clinicians or managers.

Workarounds

Viewed from a managerial perspective, it may seem that a complex socio-technical system such as a hospital functions adequately because, for the most part, the workforce complies with the policies, directives, instructions and procedures handed down from above. And this is indeed part of the story – but by no means all of it. When we examine the activities of people on the frontline of healthcare, we see that a significant proportion of their work is concerned with solving local problems in order to get the job done. This daily massaging, tweaking, compensating and adjusting is largely invisible to top management – these local fixes are what Weick has called 'dynamic non-events'. Nurses, in particular, obtain a good deal of professional satisfaction from overcoming shortcomings of the system within their wards. If a piece of equipment is missing or malfunctioning, they may 'workaround' the problem by taking a replacement from another location. But this can mean that those whose business it is to rectify the underlying organizational causes do not get to hear of these difficulties, and so an opportunity for system improvement is missed.

Tucker and Edmondson[16] observed the work of 26 nurses at nine hospitals for 239 hours. Their aim was to investigate how the corrective actions of these nurses either impeded or enhanced organizational learning from process failures. The nurses experienced five broad categories of problems: missing or incorrect information; missing or broken equipment; waiting for a human or equipment resource to appear; missing or incorrect supplies; and simultaneous demands on their time. The majority of problems crossed departmental boundaries, and most of them appeared at the safety-critical time when nurses were preparing for patient care.

On 93% of observed occasions, the nurses' problem solutions were short-term fixes that allowed them to continue caring for their patients but that did not address the underlying organizational shortcomings. Another strategy (used on 42% of occasions) was to seek help from someone close in status rather than from a more senior person who could do something about the root problem. In both cases, an opportunity for systemic improvement and organizational learning was lost.

From the nurse's immediate perspective, this first-order problem solving has much to commend it. An action is taken and the problem is gone, albeit temporarily. Moreover, these patch-up solutions enhance nurses' feelings of professional worth and are praised by their first-line supervisors. Seventy percent of the interviewed nurses said that they believed that their management expected them to work though these daily disruptions on their own. To gain attention from managers, the problem had to be one that was to be beyond the capacity of the nurse to solve by him or herself. Over time, however, the apparent balance of this approach is shown to be illusory. The system does not improve, and the problems keep recurring on a daily basis. Nurses experience an increasing sense of frustration and chronic exhaustion. As one nurse said, 'I'm quite burned out as a whole with nursing. I would quit tomorrow if I could find decent work with health insurance – even for less pay.' (reference 16, p66).

This gradually worsening situation will not heal itself. First-order problem solving confers too many short-term benefits for it to be self-correcting. Change can only result from a determined effort to get beneath the surface of the disruptions to correct the latent systemic failures that give rise to them. This means communicating with those responsible for the problem, bringing it to managers' attention, discussing how the underlying problems can be solved, and implementing remedial actions and tracking their progress. If these efforts at second-order problem solving cause professional difficulties for the nurses, or fail to achieve any systemic improvements, these learning opportunities will be lost, perhaps irrecoverably.

The normalization of deviance

'Normalization of deviance' is a phrase coined by Diane Vaughan[17] in her account of the organizational factors that contributed to the *Challenger* space shuttle disaster in January 1986. It describes the process whereby certain defects become so commonplace and so apparently inconsequential that their risk significance is gradually downgraded so that they become mere signs of normal wear and tear. The immediate cause of the *Challenger* accident was the explosive rupture of an O-ring on the launch rocket. Erosion of the O-rings had been noted on several prior launches, but these incidents were not read by the NASA engineers as signals of danger, largely because no accident had occurred. What they had not appreciated was that the brittleness of the O-rings would be catastrophically enhanced by the unusually low temperatures prevailing at the time of the *Challenger* launch.

The same process was invoked by the Columbia Accident Investigation Board as a major contributor to the *Columbia* shuttle tragedy in January 2003.[18] Foam debris damage to the spacecraft had been observed on all 113 prior shuttle flights, but it was discounted in the prelaunch decision process as not constituting a serious risk. In the event, it was a large piece of foam, penetrating the wing structure of the spacecraft, that caused its destruction on re-entry. History had apparently repeated itself.

Pathologies that arise out of the tension between production and protection

All systems are required to keep their risks *as low as reasonably practicable –* the ALARP principle. But even healthcare institutions must do this *and still stay in business* – the ASSIB principle. In short, they are required to pursue production goals and protection (or safety) goals at the same time. This is no easy task. Not only are these two goals often in conflict, at least in the short-term, they also differ in the ease with which they can be achieved:

- The information necessary to pursue these goals is not equally compelling. Whereas data relating to production is immediate, continuous and generally unambiguous; that concerning protection often comes too late or only intermittently, it is frequently ambiguous and generally not particularly reliable – as we have seen, people are not particularly anxious to pass on bad news.
- Safety has two faces: a negative aspect that is assessed through the incidence of bad events over time; and a more hidden aspect that relates to the system's robustness, resilience and ability to cope with the hazards associated with its activities. Although the negative face is the more readily quantifiable, it relates more to moments of 'unsafety' than to the intrinsic 'safety health' of the organization and cannot be taken as a reliable indicator of resilience.
- Very few clinicians or managers receive extensive training in risk management; their expertise lies primarily in the clinical or business realms.
- It is virtually impossible to foresee all the ways in which people may come to harm.
- Although failures of protection can be very expensive, it is production that pays for protection, not the other way round.
- Awareness of the patient safety problem is a relatively recent phenomenon, and is not always evident to managers and clinicians on a daily basis. But the pressure to meet production targets is immediately apparent, and continuously reinforced by governmental and top-level directives.

It is small wonder, therefore, that attempts to pursue these two aims simultaneously create at least two systemic pathologies. Each has its own unique drivers, but common to both of them is the natural ascendancy of production over protection goals. If there is a single phrase that covers both of these problems, it is 'forgetting to be afraid'. This lapse of vigilance is a direct consequence of blame and denial. Lacking reliable data about the true nature of the dangers, those who manage the institution feel safe. There may be the occasional bad apple, but the system itself is in good shape.

Trading off improved protection for increasing production

Every now and again, devices are created that offer greatly improved safety within a particular sphere of activity. Sometimes, but not always, these improved defences follow a series of bad events that have a common aetiology. In the early 19th century, for example, many coal miners had died as the result of explosions due to the insidious build up of gas and coal dust in the deeper seams. In 1815, Sir Humphry Davy invented the safety lamp that bears his name. He used a two-layer metal gauze chimney to surround and confine the flame, thus reducing the chances of it igniting methane (coaldamp). Mine owners soon realized that the invention of the Davy lamp allowed the excavation of coal from regions previously thought too dangerous to work because of the high concentrations of combustible gases. As a result, the incidence of mine explosions rose steadily after the widespread introduction of the lamp.

Similar increases in accidents occurred after the introduction of marine radar. Ship owners and masters soon discovered that radar allowed their vessels to travel at greater speeds through crowded and confined seaways. Comparable rises in accident rates were noted after the introduction of the antilocking braking system into German taxi fleets. More recently, automated short-term collision-alerting systems have been installed into the screens of air traffic controllers. This would confer added protection against midair collisions, assuming that aircraft are still required to maintain the same vertical and horizontal separations from each other. However, commercial pressures have gradually reduced these separations, thus eroding the extra margin of safety. This process has been termed 'risk compensation' or 'risk homeostasis'.[19]

Within healthcare, the use of the pulse oximeter by anaesthetists and intensivists has greatly reduced the patient's risk of suffering brain damage or death due to a failure in the supply of oxygen. I know of no instances of risk compensation in this context, but given the relentless way in which added protection is translated into productive gain, I would be surprised if such instances did not actually exist.

The blinkered pursuit of production targets

Healthcare managers are required to juggle many balls at the same time. In addition to maintaining high clinical standards, they must also pursue the efficiency and cost-saving targets that now feature so prominently in the delivery of modern healthcare. Managing by such objectives is what professional managers are trained to do, and, not unreasonably, they feel that their performance will be judged primarily by the extent to which they achieve such goals. Unfortunately, the attainment of these goals is often in direct conflict with the safety of patients.

Dietrich Doerner at the University of Bamberg has made a lifetime study of the strengths and weaknesses of human cognition when attempting to manage complex dynamic systems.[20] He found that people tend to think in causal series rather than in interacting causal networks. While they are sensitive to the main effects of their actions along a linear path towards their goals – usually expressed as numerical indicators – they are frequently unaware of the side-effects upon the rest of the system. Similarly, people are not good at controlling processes that develop in a non-linear fashion. They almost invariably underestimate their rate of change and are constantly surprised at the outcomes. Consider the following healthcare example.[21]

Managers at a UK hospital worked hard to achieve reduced waiting lists for clinical procedures and outpatient appointments. They maximized the occupancy of beds and also reduced the waiting times for treatment in the accident and emergency department. On these and other numerical indicators, the hospital was regarded as a good performer by the regional health authority. However, senior clinicians from many departments were becoming increasingly worried about the high labour turnover among the nursing staff, blood bank technicians and operating theatre assistants. They informed the management that unless action was taken very soon, the continuing loss of experienced staff would eventually paralyse the system. But the management's over-riding concern with meeting efficiency targets meant that the long-term effects of the high staff turnover were not acted upon.

The hospital's over-reliance on agency nurses resulted in decreased nursing experience on the wards. Many of the agency nurses were unfamiliar with the hospital's culture, policies, shift handover procedures and team practices. An audit by the infection control team found numerous failures by the nursing staff to comply with infection control directives and an increase in the rate of nosocomial infections. Resource shortages in the blood bank and among operating theatre assistants meant that surgical procedures had to be cancelled at short notice because the blood could not be cross-matched in time or because there was insufficient technical support available. There was also an increase in the incidence of cross-matching errors that was linked to the long hours and the poor shift patterns worked by the laboratory staff.

Examples of this relentless striving for goals that conflict with safety can be found in many hazardous domains. Perhaps the most bizarre case occurred in the Royal Navy of the mid-19th century. With the transition from sail to steam, naval officers were faced with the problem of what to do with the many sailors no longer required to rig, furl and mend sails. Their solution was to create the cult of 'brightwork' in which ships vied with one another to produce the shiniest surfaces and the glossiest paintwork. Massive watertight doors were lifted from their hinges and filed and rubbed until they gleamed – and soon lost their watertightness, a fact that cost dearly in the loss of all hands on HMS *Camperdown*.

The 20th-century record of maritime disasters also contains many instances of the single-minded but misguided pursuit of excellence contributing to catastrophic accidents. Examples range from the *Titanic* being driven at full speed into forecasted icebergs in order to clock up a transatlantic crossing record, to the capsize of the *Herald of Free Enterprise* just outside Zeebrugge in 1986. In the latter case, the shore-based managers had made their shareholders very happy in the preceding months by winning the stiff commercial competition for cross-Channel passengers; but in so doing they fatally eroded the slim safety margins on these already capsize-prone ferries.

To many hospital managers, unsafe healthcare may appear a contradiction in terms. Health and safety are two sides of the same coin; they go together. If your business is to reduce the harm caused by injury or sickness, it is easy to assume that safety is something that just emerges as a natural product of that process. But it is not. Like any other healthcare process, maintaining a high level of patient safety needs training, planning and a high level of vigilance. Above all, it needs a 'collective mindfulness' of the threats to patient safety and a continuing respect for these ever-present hazards.

The gradations of change

There are many steps along the road to attaining a safe culture, and many opportunities for failure. At any one time, a system may be in any of the states set out below. This list represents a continuum of progress along the path of change. Of the eight change conditions described, only the last involves a successful and enduring transition. Where does your organization lie on this continuum?

1. *Don't accept the need for change.* System managers are happy with the status quo. They do not believe that they have a patient safety problem. They are pleased with the way they are achieving their cost-saving and efficiency targets.
2. *Accept the need for change, but don't know where to go.* Concern has been aroused by a series of patient safety incidents. There is adverse media comment. Existing safety measures are recognized as inadequate, but the cultural deficiencies are not appreciated.
3. *Know where to go, but don't know how to get there.* It is acknowledged that the defences, barriers and controls are less than adequate. It is recognized that the organizational culture is not conducive to patient safety, but there is uncertainty about how to make the necessary improvements.
4. *Know how to get there, but doubt whether the organization can afford it.* The current new build project has over-run its budget. There is a high turnover of skilled labour and nursing shortages.

5. *Make changes, but do them only cosmetically.* Take short cuts. Fail to validate the process. Fail to monitor progress.
6. *Make changes, but no good comes of them.* The model for the changed organization does not align with the real world.
7. *The model aligns today but not tomorrow.* The change achieves only limited benefits due to unforeseen changes in the external world.
8. *Successful transition.* The changed organization keeps in step with a dynamic world and brings sustained benefit.

(I am grateful to John Wreathall for his collaboration in compiling this list.)

Conclusions

This chapter has focused far more upon describing barriers to cultural change than upon offering ways to overcome them. But there are no easy remedies for error myths and obstructive organizational dynamics. Each serves adaptive purposes for powerful individuals within the system. Identifying and acknowledging these obstacles is at least half the battle. The following points are some guidelines for improving the safety culture of healthcare systems. Adopting these precepts will not necessarily remove the organizational barriers to change, but they are an essential first step.

1. *Cease treating errors as a moral issue.* Fallibility is the norm, not the exception. There are many pressures upon doctors to bury their errors and to hide them both from their students and from the lay public. This creates the impression that only bad doctors make bad errors. But one of the basic rules of human error is that the best people can make the worst mistakes. And it is in the nature of medical practice that these errors can damage vulnerable people. This is a circumstantial issue, not a moral one.
2. *Understand that errors do not inevitably lead to adverse events.* Many experienced healthcare professionals possess the ability to detect and recover their errors before they do harm – although, for the most part, this is a skill acquired through bitter experience rather than formal training. But its basics – vigilance and mindfulness of danger – can also be taught.
3. *Like aviators, always take human fallibility as a given.* Many flying instructors, for example, will not let their students go solo until they have made a shaky landing and recovered from it. Once healthcare professionals acknowledge their fallibility, they can begin to accept the need for gaining the personal and practical skills necessary to cope with the certainty of error and with its recovery.

4. *Recognize that errors are consequences rather than causes.* They are not simply the product of incompetence, mental waywardness or perversity. The immediate psychological precursors of error – inattention, preoccupation, distraction or forgetfulness – are often the last and least manageable part of a much longer story that extends back to the working conditions, the system at large and, perhaps most importantly, to the organizational and professional culture.

5. *Appreciate that while it may be emotionally satisfying (and legally and managerially convenient) to name, blame and shame those who make errors, this common reaction has little or no remedial value.* In the first place, it isolates the individual from his or her systemic context – thus preventing the identification and removal of error-provoking features of the workplace. Second, such an approach carries the assumption that only bad people make errors. Of course, there are egregious errors, even in medicine. But these comprise only a very small proportion of all the errors made. We can only learn about situational error traps if people report their errors and near-misses.

6. *Design healthcare systems for real human beings – with all their failings – rather than for some angelic and omniscient ideal.* This means creating error-tolerant systems that anticipate, detect, forgive and recover errors. Everyday word-processing packages can achieve this, so why not healthcare institutions? Simple ergonomic good practice would be a start: standardization, good illumination, legible script, sensible working hours and the like. At the moment, many operating theatres – to take just one example – are little short of ergonomic nightmares. Because healthcare institutions do not always acknowledge the likelihood of errors, they fail to take adequate countermeasures. Because doctors are reared in the illusion of infallibility, they are prepared to work under conditions that would have made a 19th century factory owner blush; indeed, they often take it as a mark of pride. That attitude may have been well suited to a First World War casualty clearing station, but it is wholly inappropriate for high-technology healthcare facilities in the 21st century.

7. *Finally, understand that when adverse events happen and patients are harmed, the victims and their relatives want four things: an acknowledgement that an error was made, an acceptance of responsibility, a sincere apology and an assurance that the lessons learned from this mishap will help to prevent its recurrence.* The need for financial compensation may arise when the harm caused requires it, but it is not the general rule. The fear of litigation does not have to be an insuperable barrier to effective error management.

References

1. Vincent C, Neale G, Woloshynowych M. Adverse events in British hospitals: preliminary retrospective record review. *BMJ* 2001; **322:** 517–19.
2. Davis P, Lay-Yee R, Briant R, Ali W *et al.* Adverse events in New Zealand public hospitals 1: occurrence and impact. *NZ Med J* 2002; **115:** U271.
3. Schioler T, Lipczak H, Pedersen BL *et al.* Danish Adverse Event Study. [Incidence of adverse events in hospitals. A retrospective study of medical records.] *Ugeskr Laeger* 2001; **163:** 5370–8.
4. Thomas EJ, Studdert DM, Runciman WB *et al.* A comparison of iatrogenic injury studies in Australia and the USA. 1: Context, methods, casemix, population, patient and hospital characteristics. *Int J Qual Health Care* 2000; **12:** 371–8.
5. Baker RG, Norton PG, Flintoft V *et al.* The Canadian Adverse Events Study: the incidence of adverse events among hospital patients in Canada. *CMAJ* 2004; **17:** 1678–86.
6. QuIC. Doing What Counts for Patient Safety. *Summary of the Report to the President of the Quality Interagency Coordination Task Force.* Washington, DC: QuIC, 2000.
7. Reason J. *Human Error.* New York: Academic Press, 1990.
8. Mach, E. *Knowledge and Error.* Dordrecht: Reidel, 1905 [English translation, 1976].
9. Amalberti R, Wioland L. Human error in aviation. In: Soekkha HM (ed) *Aviation Safety.* Utrecht: VSP, 1997: 91–100.
10. de Leval M, Carthey J, Wright D *et al.* Human factors and cardiac surgery: a multicentre study. *J Thorac Cardiovasc Surg* 2000; **119:** 661–72.
11. Weick KE, Sutcliffe KM, Obstfeld D. Organising for high reliability processes of collective mindfulness. *Res Organis Behav* 1999; **21:** 23–81.
12. Reason J. *Managing the Risks of Organisational Accidents.* Aldershot: Ashgate, 1997.
13. Westrum R. A typology of organisational cultures. *Qual Safety Health Care* 2004; **13**(Suppl II): ii22–7.
14. Weick KE, Sutcliffe KM. Hospitals as cultures of entrapment: a re-analysis of the Bristol Royal Infirmary. *Calif Manag Rev* 2003; **45:** 73–84.
15. Morrison EW, Milliken FJ. Organisational silence: a barrier to change and development in a pluralistic world. *Acad Manag Rev* 2000; **25:** 708–725.
16. Tucker AL, Edmondson AC. Why hospitals don't learn from failures: organisational and psychological dynamics that inhibit system change. *Calif Manag Rev* 2003; **45:** 55–72.
17. Vaughan D. *The Challenger Launch Decision: Risky Technology, Culture and Deviance at NASA.* Chicago: University of Chicago Press, 1996.
18. *The Columbia Accident Investigation Report.* Washington, DC: National Aeronautics and Space Administration and Government Printing Office, August 2003.
19. Wilde GJS. The theory of risk homeostasis: implications for safety and health. *Risk Anal* 1982; **2:** 209–55.
20. Doerner D. *The Logic of Failure.* New York: Metropolitan Books, 1996.
21. Reason J, Carthey J, de Leval MR. Diagnosing 'vulnerable system syndrome': an essential prerequisite to effective risk management. *Qual Health Care* 2001; **10**(Supp II): ii21–5.

2

Fixing the broken triangle: Improving patient and public involvement in clinical governance, locally and nationally

Bob Sang

'All "clinical governance complaints" (save those which do not involve serious issues of patient safety and where the underlying facts giving rise to the complaint are clear and undisputed) should be referred to the inter-PCT investigation team. The objects of the investigation should be to reach a conclusion as to what happened and to set out the evidence and conclusions in a report which should go to **the PCT with responsibility for the doctor**. If the investigators are unable to reach a conclusion about what happened because there is an unresolved conflict of evidence, they should say so in their report.'

[My emphasis] (Reference 1 Report 5, Recommendation 9, Paragraph 27.50)

The above, unequivocal, recommendation from the Shipman Inquiry[1] endorses a fundamental principal of quality management: namely, that improvement starts and ends 'at source'. In this chapter, I wish to relate the current debate about professional accountability in healthcare, including the consideration of the role of national bodies such as the General Medical Council (GMC), with the local implementation of clinical governance. The Shipman Inquiry has been reporting at a time when new legislation is being implemented that requires that all local boards, such as Primary Care Trust (PCT) boards, carry responsibility for clinical governance and for ensuring meaningful, appropriate and effective patient and public involvement in decision making, monitoring, and public scrutiny. But, what does this mean in practice and for practice, at national and local levels? In particular, how can we develop the means to ensure continuous improvement that are constructive for doctors and other clinicians?

Once the findings of the Shipman Inquiry have been fully considered and consulted upon, a fresh, open and rigorous approach must be developed that patients, practitioners, and the wider public can trust. This chapter endeavours to offer a basis for such a system of governance and regulation in healthcare.

Introduction

Transforming regulatory assumptions

'Context is (almost) everything'[2]

There is a deep and deepening ambiguity associated with defining people by their state of ill health and consequent use of health and care services arising from the twin ideological forces of consumerism ('Patient Choice') and citizenship (peoples' responsibilities). Concurrently, the essential nature of professionalism and the regulation of healthcare professions is being challenged. The evolving theory and practice of medicine, and its contribution to well-being at every level – personal, family, community, economic and civic – are converging with the social and cultural redefinitions of what it means to be a 'patient' or 'service user'. The 'lay' view is subject to surveys, media interpretations and conjecture: with many interest groups claiming to represent patients' interests. Those working in the field of public engagement are beginning to question the value and relevance of 'representation' as a model of promoting involvement, recognizing that people can speak for themselves. So how might their voices contribute to improving clinical governance at the core of professional regulation in healthcare?

The challenges to established cultures from these new ways of working are growing, with concurrent implications for the leadership and regulation of the medical profession. What can be learned from other domains of public and community engagement, or from the re-regulation of other similar professions such as nursing and social work? And, if there is an institutional failure to learn, what might be the consequences for doctors, for patients and for public trust?

When exploring the meaning and purpose of public involvement and engagement, it is always worth asking potential participants 'What's in it for you/me/us?' What motivates people to involve themselves in the structures and processes of others – to engage in the business of medical regulation and leadership? And, are the reasons to engage good enough in the systems of modern healthcare and their increasingly dynamic context? In an era when growing numbers of people develop a long-term relationship with their local and specialist healthcare services as a result of chronic disease and disability, gaining real insight into the interactions between medicine and society at every level, it is important to consider how such assets can contribute to improving medical practice and the governance of the profession. After all, 'We are all in this together'.[3]

Role conflict or synergy?

'We want to be treated as whole people with whole lives'[4]

'Sick' people have many roles – neighbour, friend, parent, partner, employee, carer – as do professionals. In healthcare, everyone has potential conflicts of interest and, in a resource-rich yet financially restricted system, there is always competition. 'Patterns of dominance' have evolved around the competition for resources, with many claiming 'public interest' as their competitive advantage. Could public involvement in clinical governance and medical regulation, as well as in the development of the profession itself, be based on sufficient common purpose to transcend the inherent conflicts and tensions?

There are a number of important aspects of this challenge:

- *Expertise*: 'Lay' people bring their own expertise and experiences of disease and disability – a complement to medical knowledge and practice. Consequently, services' improvement and governance have the potential to become a genuinely collaborative endeavour.
- *Ideology*: The medical model is increasingly at odds with the social and civic models of care and participation in health systems. Might a more potent synthesis be developed that will help regulators and clinical evaluators address the issues of public accountability and professional leadership with which they are being confronted?
- *Proportionality*: 'Whose majority is it anyway?' What can be learned from bodies where patients/users/citizens form the majority of the governing bodies (e.g. in the disability and social care spheres). Will the medical profession be willingly led by the 'laity'? How might this work at a local level, in trusts, PCTs and in general practice.
- *Citizenship*: 'Label jars, not people'.[5] Is the work of the GMC, the 'think tanks', interested academics and active patients producing a concept of 'good citizen' that reflects the wisdom, sensitivity and public spirit that can be brought by all contributors to the engagement process? Following some years of experimentation, are we creating a model of engagement that transcends labels and spurious 'representativeness' that could be adopted by regulatory bodies in implementing their public duties and regulatory tasks? Is such task-focused public engagement a useful complement to formal clinical governance arrangements locally and nationally – reducing the load on committees and producing evidence, advice and findings through robust, transparent, temporary processes? And, where is the 'critical friend' in the governance system itself – ensuring that the professions do not end up talking to themselves? Could temporary working groups – 'loose gangs' (Catto) – be formed to address specific public interest issues: assess the

evidence, feedback and close (e.g. in relation to service redesign and referral changes)?

Improving the regulatory dialogue – Is shared clinical governance desirable/possible?

Doctors are bright people who are in the business of dealing with human complexity: biological, emotional, psychological and socio-cultural. Marginalize them, or condemn them to mundanity, and they develop a capacity for mischief making and worse. Patients, in all their diversity, are the primary source of the complexity addressed by doctors and they provide a continuing challenge to the limits of medical knowledge. Traditionally, doctors have dealt with such complexity in their own systems (peer review, etc.) and patients have created their own complex system of organizations, ranging from overt campaigning lobby groups to competing service organizations. As fellow citizens, doctors and patients confront this challenge both personally ('people are learning to change themselves') and collectively (co-creation, co-determination and even co-regulation). Enlightened self-interest and civic engagement fuse uncomfortably to undermine traditional models of self-referential, self-preserving professional leadership and the consequent historically dependent behaviours of citizens. Building mutual confidence and trust is a matter of exploration, discovery, dialogue and critical review – a critique that takes regulation well beyond peer assessment and 'lay' participation in committee structures towards modes of engagement that will require imaginative ways of 'filling the empty chair'. 'Loose gangs' of practitioners, patients and skilled enablers could be commissioned to address the complex issues that now confront medical practice: from ethical dilemmas, to errors and dysfunctionality, to redesigning protocols and standards. Continuous innovation and development could beget continuous engagement: purposeful, meaningful and appropriate engagement of busy people with complex lives – lives that are often under stress, lives where nurturing (not blame) and mutual endeavour produces helpful outcomes. How might such 'mutuality' work in the day-to-day practice of clinical governance?

Patient involvement in clinical governance: involving to improve

'Patient and Public Involvement in Health' (PPIH) is now enshrined in legislation[6] and the proposed 'Patient Focus' standards of the new Healthcare

Commission. This section reflects their significance and, by drawing on the principles of continuous quality improvement (CQI), offers some practical advice on taking forward patient involvement in clinical governance.

The new 'patient-centred' context: 'nothing about me without me'

First and foremost, we need a much more robust and less rhetorical analysis of 'patient-focused patient-centredness', and, of course, patients themselves have a great deal to say on the subject. Analysis shows us just how much the patient movement has matured in the UK in the modern era:

- There now exists 25 years' experience of developing and supporting independent lay advocacy, working with our most vulnerable fellow citizens. Hundreds of local schemes, supported by national enabling networks, recruit and train local citizens to participate effectively in achieving healthier lives.[7]
- The Consumers Advisory Group on Clinical Trials has helped to lead the way in involving patients in primary medical research.[8]
- The Disability Movement and 'Expert Patient' initiative, led by the Long-Term Medical Conditions Alliance, have taken our understanding of patient self-determination and the self-management of disease to a much higher level.
- The College of Health's 'Voices In Action' programme, funded by the Department of Health, has involved a wide range of service users in the development of excellent training materials for lay representatives.[9]
- The King's Fund and Institute of Public Policy Research have successfully demonstrated that 'ordinary wisdom works': i.e., through such means as Citizens' juries, lay people can take on tough health policy decisions, including handling contentious or even contradictory medical evidence.[10]
- Finally, the Commission for Patient and Public Involvement in Health supports direct patient involvement in the 'community governance' of the NHS by aligning patients' groups with PCTs and NHS trust boards, monitored by local patient and public involvement forums (PPIFs) and local government health overview and scrutiny committees (under Sections 7 and 11 of the 2001 Health and Social Care Act).

However, at a local level, the development of the patient 'voice' and meaningful patient participation is still patchy and uneven. In this context, how might we ensure that patient involvement in clinical governance is both appropriate and effective – everywhere?

The core principles: towards inclusive and effective clinical governance

I would like to suggest an approach that is grounded in three principles, namely *informed dialogue, triangulation* and *shared learning about risk*, supported organizationally by a commitment to continuous learning, innovation and improvement – the CQI approach. In the spirit of CQI, 'patient-centred' means an open reciprocal approach to clinical governance that fosters mutual respect and demonstrable health benefits.

Informed dialogue

In the past, most attempts to involve patients on the development and governance of clinical services have been *ad hoc*, reactive, and provider-driven: often taking the provision of information for granted. However, recent literature on the subject gives us a useful evaluation of a wide range of methods of achieving lay participation in health systems.[11,12] And, as we have noted above, we are gaining valuable experience from working with patients in primary clinical research as well as in the planning and development of services. But, governance is distinctively concerned with assuring measurable accountability for personal, team and organizational performance. All participants in a governance process can learn to understand the significance of this responsibility and how to obtain, use and assess pertinent information. In so doing, they need to ensure they have a meaningful dialogue and develop mutual understanding. Without this, we risk implementing clinical governance that is partial and potentially compromised – both for clinicians and for patients. There are two kinds of information that matter: *process information* (the values and objectives that validate a robust, fair approach to clinical governance) and *substantive information* (concerned with disease and clinical practice and the evidence base that allows us to assess clinical effectiveness). How can we enable patients and clinicians to have and to share sufficient mastery of both forms of information?

Triangulation

We firmly believe that the clinical governance process will not achieve the performance outcomes and wider public legitimacy it deserves unless we validate evidence of clinical practitioner, team and organizational performance from three complementary perspectives: those of professional peers, of clinical and service team partners (whether inside or outside the organization), *and* of patients.

Clearly, this is an aspect of development that will be enriched by a great deal of innovation as colleagues gain confidence in opening up their clinical performance for wider scrutiny. It is worth reminding ourselves that excellent practitioners have developed this habit of triangulation as a means of continuously improving their knowledge and practice as a virtuous cycle.[13] From listening assiduously to patients and colleagues, to reflecting out loud with larger groups, and through dissemination, excellent practitioners test themselves through formal and informal triangulation on a daily basis. Our challenge is to make this habit more systematic in an even more helpful way, and in ways that the public can trust.

Sharing learning about risk

Modern medicine, and public attitudes about medicine, are still bedevilled by a mythology about the absolute quality of medical knowledge, the perfectibility of the human condition and the achievement of risk-free healthcare. We often share a 'mutual expectation deficit', which enables us to avoid talking about the reality of the risks that exist in all that we do, whether in daily life or in clinical practice. Every patient is different, and access to the medical knowledge base is growing fast – often, however, it does so unreliably for personal and organizational reasons. A mature relationship between clinicians and patients (and/or their advocates) is based on a process of learning – an exploration that is informed by the available evidence, the exercise of judgement and the process of diagnosis itself. Cancer patients have developed the notion of 'the patient's journey' – a concept that is now more widely used across the patient movement to explain patients' understanding of the gaps and connections in service, as well as the unpredictability of challenging disease from an individual patient's point of view. If we are all to be valued partners in these journeys, then our ability to be open about the risks, including being clear about our own uncertainties and lack of knowledge, is critical to achieving the cultural change that will sustain an effective and trusted system of clinical governance.[14]

So, how can we approach such a challenge sensitively and practically? Our colleagues from patients' organizations understand the strategic nature both of the clinical governance agenda and of the importance of working cooperatively and incrementally, building on small 'early' successes and sharing learning about improving practice. This is about managing innovation and making it stick – the essence of a continuous quality improvement approach.[15]

The conceptual underpinning of CQI in health: meaningful, purposeful triangulation

Patient involvement in clinical governance adds important dimensions both to the rigour of the clinical governance process itself and to the potential for learning on all sides – a model of triangulation that builds up to a powerful tool for whole system improvement reflecting the principles of CQI developed above.

CQI has emerged in other sectors for three principal reasons:

- Because it is not programmatic, it can be developed flexibly as external forces change and new 'business' needs emerge.
- It is inherently 'customer-driven', enabling organizations to respond continuously to feedback from their users/clients.
- It promotes learning and continuous development of staff at all levels in the organization, including the board.

Thus, in health, patients become the 'drivers' of CQI as much as individual healthcare professionals and teams.

The focus of clinical governance is the individual practitioner and relationships between team and patient: i.e. it is a 'systems' approach, linking day-to-day practice to the changing circumstances of the services and the communities it services. By involving her/his peers, their service partners in the whole clinical process (nurses, p.a.m.s, social care, therapists) and patients themselves, we can create three domains for personal development and learning: this is the principle of triangulation (Figure 2.1).

Implementation of this core framework will produce a multidisciplinary and multiagency approach to clinical governance that informs integrated pathways: *the patient's journey.* It will also, critically, stimulate shared learning with patients and the clinical community. This feeds organizational learning in the process: the second learning loop, linking *patients' experiences* directly to the development of services and the multidisciplinary staff who work with them (Figure 2.2).

So, how might these frameworks be put to use in healthcare settings?

Towards effective implementation: mapping, communicating, networking

If patients are really to be central in this process, then it is important to think about involving them from the outset. Thus, an important preliminary step is to identify the patients and advocacy groups active in your NHS Trust or wider

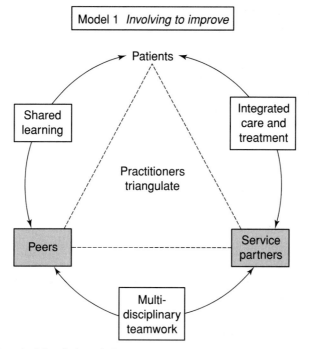

FIGURE 2.1 The principle of triangulation.

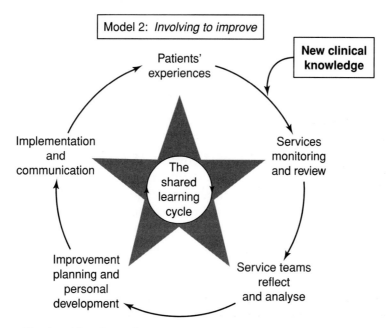

FIGURE 2.2 The shared learning cycle

health economy, and to analyse the nature of their engagement. In parallel, clinical and management colleagues may be actively working with patients on a range of activities: from research and development through service innovations, to monitoring and evaluation. Such a 'mapping' exercise can be assessed according to a number of criteria, principally:

- Is it patient-led, clinician-led or a joint approach?
- How well are patients informed about (a) process and (b) priorities, standards, and evidence?
- Is the process temporary or continuous?
- Are the means of involvement standardized (e.g. pre-designed questionnaires) or participatory (e.g. focus groups) – formal or informal? Are they *independently* supported?
- Is the focus strategic or operational?

Then:

- What is being achieved (including mistakes and misjudgements)?
- What is being learned (by whom and how)? Or not?
- What can improve (taking note of the criteria elaborated above) when it is done again?
- How are the answers to the above questions communicated, and to whom?

In sum, such an analysis can complement and enhance the baseline assessment produced during the first stages of the implementation of clinical governance. It is worth taking time on this initial work, and then identifying two or three projects where patients can be explicitly involved in improving clinical practice and, in the process, contributing to the improvement of clinical governance. Such a participatory approach necessarily entails a synthesis of qualitative and quantitative methods[11,12] and designing an action research approach that complements and supports sound clinical research. We envisage that patient involvement in clinical governance will increasingly stimulate enrichment of both the delivery of clinical services and our knowledge of the use and experience of clinical services and technologies. An exciting prospect and a key dimension to governance is a partnership that negotiates the balance of power within the healthcare system – especially when learning is networked across and between local health economies. Indeed, as we share learning about the development of inclusive and effective clinical governance, and as we implement clinical networks themselves, so we will begin to realize the vision of a truly 'relationship-centred' NHS.

Conclusion: fixing the broken triangle – involving patients and the public in the regulation of healthcare practice

Redefining the challenge

CQI occurs locally, inclusively and incrementally. So, how might we translate local improvement into a regulated, contentious, national context? Commentators have rightly distinguished between 'public' and 'patient' interests in the regulation of clinical practice.

Consider Figure 2.3. 'Triangulation' is also the essence of robust regulation: the development of systems of accountability that integrate public protection, professional/practitioners' peer review and patient experience. It is not good enough for the self-referential institutions of practice to claim 'patients' best interests', nor at present are the public systems of monitoring and scrutiny adequate; likewise, the systems of providing patient information and representation are variable and often self-serving.

As indicated above, credible public and patient involvement in regulation will be grounded in *local* systems of clinical governance and quality assurance that, in turn, inform the development of the curriculum and the standards and processes of accreditation and revalidation. The effectiveness of the role of the regulator as leader, enabler and ultimate adjudicator is dependent on

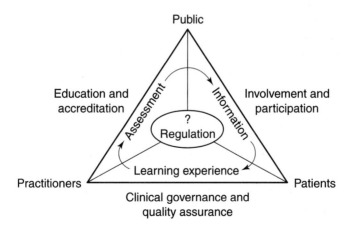

FIGURE 2.3 A virtuous triangle?

clarification of these processes and on successful transfer of the evidence for improvement between their interfaces.

Further, the regulator is dependent for its success as much on the work of those responsible for facilitating active, informed, citizenship in health, as on the relevance and reliability of national *and* local quality assurance systems (e.g. the NHS Performance Management and Quality Assurance System).

In reality, the situation is less clear-cut: the triangle is actually stretched apart in all its sides, with the major 'pull' forces most evident at the apexes. The cause of this 'stretch' is that the key tasks (assessment, information, learning) have been evolving in parallel, separated by institutional assumptions of power, control, and authority (Figure 2.4).

In a culture that is increasingly being driven by patients themselves, these assumptions are becoming a less acceptable influence on the dynamic flow of the system. However, the current reforms in patient and public involvement in health (see above) will do little to reverse the pull effect of the contending institutional interests at the apexes, for the following reasons:

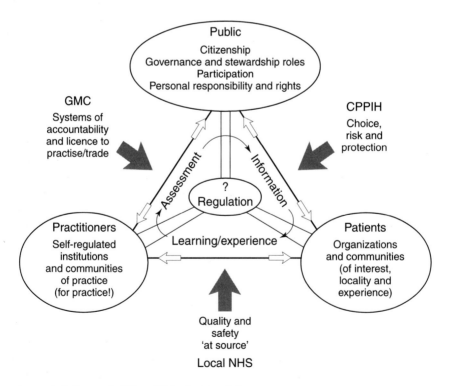

FIGURE 2.4 Pull or push: Who will fix the triangle?

- *Citizenship* is underinvested and confused.
- *Patients* remain subject to profound inequalities.
- *Practitioners* are highly self-protective and remain economically and culturally powerful, despite attempts to impose managerial systems (e.g. the new contracts for GPs and consultants).
- The supply of information is subject to powerful vested interests in a highly complex, increasing technological set of drivers (e.g. digital TV, e-empowerment).

How might future regulators both impact on and influence this increasingly dynamic scenario?

Fixing the triangle: showing the way in modern medicine

Trust is the glue

Practitioner-led regulation does not work on its own. Patients need to have confidence that their feedback (positive and negative) has a demonstrable effect. There needs to be proper public scrutiny of the processes of assessment, accountability, and (re)validation/accreditation. And, in the 'third chair', there needs to be a means of ensuring civic overview of the processes of information, fair redress and public scrutiny.

Tokenism is worse than doing nothing

Until now the GMC, the Royal Colleges and other regulators have worked both through their own structures and through relationships with national bodies such as the Patients Association. In quality assurance terms, they have responded to patients' concerns through 'exception reporting' mechanisms, such as complaints and investigations. Feedback into curriculum reform is painstaking and bureaucratic, lagging behind some of the other professions in respect of active user/patient involvement, rendering grassroots clinical governance ineffective as a means of sustainable improvement.

In order to build public confidence and patient trust, an implementation strategy is called for that demonstrably impacts in four key domains:

1. *Quick and fair redress* when things go wrong (note that this 'bottom-line' requirement crucially depends on the local management of complaints, Patient Advice and Liaison Service (PALS), Independent Complaints Advocacy Service (ICAS), and direct public concerns, necessitating a good mutual understanding between local boards, the GMC and the Healthcare Commission).

2. *Advice and agreements on the inputs and outputs* of clinical governance systems, building on the 'involving to improve' models (above).
3. *An overarching agreement* with the NHS Healthcare Commission and CPPIH on goals, roles, rules and boundaries for local monitoring and scrutiny.
4 *Impact on the content and design* of the medical education curriculum, including demonstrable participation of patients in the delivery and assessment of medical education – from first-year undergraduates to ongoing personal and professional development.

Patients and the public can be involved in establishing the parameters of each of the above domains – but not necessarily through the existing structures and processes.

Citizens become involved for a good purpose. As we found with Citizens' Juries, it is good to involve people on a serious, time-limited task whereby the results of their involvement can be put to demonstrable good use. Standing groups, committees and councils can become rapidly detached from the day-to-day experience of patients unless they are enriched by such constructive, temporary processes of involvement – collaboratively designed and independently facilitated.[10]

A fresh approach is called for: a way forward for clinical governance locally, and professional regulation nationally?

Acknowledgement

This chapter is based on an article written with Steve O'Neill, 'Patient involvement in clinical governance', which appeared in the *British Journal of Healthcare Management* (2001; **7**: 7). I am very grateful to Professor Sir Graeme Catto and Harry Cayton, OBE, for their encouragement and the opportunity to reflect constructively on these issues. Indeed, the learning from such interventions can be networked, through real and virtual means, facilitated by an independent host, sponsored by a collaborative of professionals, patients, and regulators – 'Nothing about us, without us'.

References

1. The Shipman Inquiry, Fifth Report. *Safeguarding Patients: Lessons from the Past – Proposals for the Future*. Command Paper Cm 6394, 9 December 2004.
2. Sang B, Maclenahan J. *Health at Work*. London: HEA, 1999.

3. *The Future of Access to General Practice-based Primary Medical Care Informing the Debate*. Review paper prepared for the Royal College of General Practitioners and the NHS Alliance. London: Royal College of General Practitioners, 2004.
4. *Citizens Voices Report*. London: King's Fund, 1998.
5. *People First*, 1982.
6. *Strengthening Accountability*. London: Department of Health, March 2003.
7. Clements J, Sang B. Voices of difference. *J Health Law* 2000.
8. *Involvement Works: 2nd Report of the Standing Advisory Group on Consumer Involvement in NHS Research*. London: Department of Health 1999.
9. Bradburn J, Fletcher G, Kennelly C. *Voices in Action*. London: College of Health, 2002.
10. Elizabeth S, Sang B, Hanley B. *Ordinary Wisdom*. London: King's Fund, 1999.
11. Chambers R. *Involving Patients and the Public*. Oxford: Radcliffe Medical Press, 2000.
12. Barker J, DeVille J, Bullen M. *Reference Manual for Public Involvement*. London: Department of Health, 1999.
13. Brockbank A, McGill I. *Facilitating Reflective Learning*. Milton Keynes: Open University Press, 1999.
14. Sang B, Keep J, Cowper A. Choice, Risk and Accountability. *J Healthcare Manag* December 2004.
15. Bessant J. *High Involvement Innovation*. Chichester: Wiley, 2004.

3 Organizational culture: Cultural indicators as a tool for performance improvement

Rosemary Hittinger and L Peter Fielding

Introduction

> 'Culture is a body of learned behavior, a collection of beliefs, habits, practices and traditions shared by a group of people and successfully learned by new members who enter the society.'
>
> Margaret Mead[1]

Over the last 50 years, the increasing complexity of medicine and the means of its delivery through healthcare systems has become one of society's most pressing problems because of the ever-expanding treatment options for patient care and because of its ever-increasing real costs. In addition, the decline in manpower recruitment for most healthcare professions is a social phenomenon in many countries (including the UK and North America), which makes the smooth delivery of efficient services a great challenge. In parallel, there has been an increased demand for higher levels of social accountability from those who provide these healthcare services. Failure to recognize these new professional and social circumstances, at a time of increased exposure of both physician and system failures, has resulted in a substantial loss of confidence in the medical profession.[2-4] This fundamental change in the relationship between society and the medical profession has permeated all levels from national and regional government to local healthcare serve provider units, and even to the level of individual doctor–patient consultation.

Although there has been some recognition within the medical profession of these societal changes in recent years, this has been more apparent in central bureaucracy than in the medical profession's behaviour. Indeed, a bunker mentality to mount a rearguard action to preserve the old 'club culture'[5, 6] remains common, however obliquely expressed. The profession must now make a fundamental decision – either to blame outside agencies for the current difficulties as an act of self-justification, or to become more transparent and accountable for the medicine that is practised and the outcomes that are achieved.

The complexity of modern medicine demands that methods be used to recognize the effects of confounding variables as we study clinical outcome. Equally, however, it must be recognized that errors and near-misses occur too frequently[3] and great variations in clinical methods and outcomes are the norm rather than the exception.[7, 8]

Unfortunately, this choice is no longer a free one. Society is now demanding, through governmental bodies, the establishment of targets, clinical performance indicators and other mechanisms aimed at achieving a high degree of accountability and control over the medical profession. The imposition of these targets is, in part, a consequence of the profession's lack of timely response to the excessive clinical outcome variances that have been so widely exposed in the media.

It is in this context that healthcare professionals of all types are being asked to treat their patients in a safe, timely, effective, efficient, equitable and patient-centred (STEEP) fashion.[4, 9] In addition, it is reasonable that patients should wish these professional attributes to be provided in a personable, positive and pleasant style.

We call the local micro-environments in which people interact to display these beneficial qualities a 'positive medical culture' (PMC).

Thus, the purpose of this chapter is to provide a framework for both the creation and assessment of a PMC in an optimistic environment in which *people care for people*. Although the culture of an organization may seem intangible, we suggest that by observing certain features of structure and behaviour, by asking the right questions and by reviewing certain documents, a picture emerges of what we can call its 'culture'.[10] We are convinced that for a PMC to thrive, we must achieve a respectful, committed and truthful culture, all of which are central to the delivery of predictable and high-performance healthcare.[11]

These activities are often grouped under the general title of 'clinical governance' in the UK and of 'performance improvement' in the USA, but the intention is the same – namely to provide the vision, code of conduct and theoretical underpinnings to cradle the conflicts that are intrinsic to the process of performance improvement.[12] The embedded notion of quality improvement in healthcare provision depends on the development of an appropriate cultural reference.[11]

Therefore, a robust set of 'cultural indicators' are needed to provide a tool to separate the spoken and written promises inherent in well-meaning vision statements and to distil the reality that affects so intimately the lives of all those who work in healthcare institutions and those who are treated by them.

Although a framework with its goals and objectives may be identified at the national level, implementation must be within a local community where people work, interact and create the relationships upon which healthcare provision is based.

There are many ways in which an institutional culture can be described and classified, with differing methods of grouping and dividing each topic. However, the details are less important than the general principles that we have attempted to capture in this chapter. Broadly speaking, we suggest that a PMC is one in which the staff (i.e. all those who work in healthcare, including nurses and doctors) are supported, errors and near-misses are identified, and lessons are learned within a general ethos of public service and integrity. (Such a culture has been recommended by the findings of the Bristol Inquiry.[5]) In contrast, a negative culture is one in which there is an idiosyncratic, self-serving autocracy in which problems result in arbitrary and sometimes capricious actions. Such organizations are not necessarily easy to identify, because they may contain persuasive individuals who are practised at statements of intent (where words such as 'collaboration' and 'partnership' are heavily used with ideological correctness), but where these qualities are not evidenced or observed.

Because people and relationships are at the core of healthcare delivery, we have chosen to start with human resources (HR) and staffing issues as our first indicator. This is followed by another seven indicators: policies and procedures; goals and objectives; performance indicators and physician variation; process re-engineering; risk management; the environment; and customer services. A summary of the evidence required within each category is shown in Table 3.1. We believe that this checklist will provide an objective and reproducible tool for assessing a PMC of an organization whether it is in primary, secondary or tertiary patient care.

Human resources and staffing

The number of interactions necessary for even quite simple healthcare processes can be extraordinarily large. Thus, the interaction between people should be at the core of any review of institutional culture and evidenced by the presence and usage of a comprehensive set of policies and procedures.

Recruitment

There should be an acknowledgement by HR to the effect that those recruited should be selected for their professional talent and *cultural maturity*.[13] In

TABLE 3.1 Checklist of indicators and summary of evidence required within each category

Indicator	Policy or procedure	Measurement
Human resources and staffing		
Recruitment practices	Philosophy of hiring for talent and cultural maturity	Policy present/absent
	Orientation process for all people working in the organization according to professional type	Records of attendance and by professional group
Staff evaluation	All employees have annual evaluation, including senior management	Availability of appraisal for all staff members.
		Availability of meaningful professional development plans following annual appraisal
Disciplinary procedures	Defined disciplinary procedures and evidence that they are followed	Policy present/absent, HR records of disciplinary processes, follow-ups and results
	Bullying and retaliation policy	Policy present/absent
	General harassment policy	Policy present/absent
	Disruptive behaviour policy	Policy present/absent
Staff statistics	Sickness and turnover data by department and institution	Data availability
	Exit interviews for all staff	Documentation and analysis available
Staff satisfaction surveys	Staff satisfaction survey takes place at least annually	Summary of results and action plans available
Policies and procedures		
Performance management	Clear separation of 'formative' and 'normative' processes in both structure and assessment personnel	Organizational charts that clearly identify these features
Openness and transparency	Complaints (both internal and external) will be dealt with promptly, candidly and objectively	Data maintained of complaints by unit and evidence of responses

TABLE 3.1 *continued*

Indicator	Policy or procedure	Measurement
Goals and objectives		
Departmental annual reports	Measurable outcomes and metrics of change with minutes and attendance records of monthly meetings	Reports to be available
Communication	Institution-wide means of communication	Copies to be kept on file and evidence of circulation
Physician attendance at organizational and peer review meetings	Expected percentage attendance of individual doctors accepting seats on committees	Attendance data for each committee member
Performance indicators		
Physician variance	Individual and aggregate data available for chosen study populations (high-volume and/or high-risk cases)	Data analysis and performance improvement initiatives to be documented and available
No-blame environment	Policies, procedures	Meeting minutes demonstrating this approach
Process change and re-engineering		
New ideas	Evidence that front-line staff are encouraged to contribute new ideas and process re-engineering	Maintain records of these changes and their celebration
Process review	All members of staff will set out to identify areas of work simplification	Records of process change by department or unit. Policy that new or changed process will be embedded in routine practice
	Staff encouraged to identify and remediate process bottlenecks and reduce duplicated activities	Audits of new processes to demonstrate improved efficacy and efficiency
Embedding process	Careful assessment and justification of new administrative posts that measurably demonstrates the anticipated value to the organization	Records available

Indicator	Policy or procedure	Measurement
Risk management		
Critical incident reviews	Definition of structure and function of root cause analysis and other ways that clinical incident reviews will take place	Evidence of implementation and monitoring of action plans
Database	All incidents and near-misses will be entered into a database and outcomes recorded	Evidence of timely actions and feedback to the involved parties
Environmental issues		
	Institution will be maintained in a clean and cared-for state	Direct personal visits and review
Customer service		
Surveys	Surveys of patients, staff and physicians at least annually	Evidence of usage and feedback to relevant professional groups

addition, there should be a formally constructed and regularly carried-out introduction to the organization, which should take place as part of the induction process at the start of the new employee's service. This orientation process should be for everyone joining the organization, including medical staff and senior management. Data recording the participation in this orientation should be maintained by professional discipline.

Staff evaluation

There should be evidence of annual performance appraisals for all staff grades, including nurses, doctors and management (not less than annually), with problem identification and resolution occurring within a 'blame-free' approach. Members of the relevant middle or senior management personnel in the professional area concerned should carry out each appraisal. Training is necessary for these appraisals and the format should be part standardized for the whole institution and part relative to the area in which the staff person works. There should be open responses from all those reviewed, with meaningful professional development plans that can form the basis of the following year's appraisal. Evidence of late appraisals, little or no contribution to the documentation by affected individual staff members, missing information for specific staff groupings, or a lack of evidence of development, change and improvement are all signs of a negative culture.

There must be evidence of a clear policy of zero-tolerance for bullying, retaliation, gender harassment and other forms of disruptive behaviour. Not only is it important to have such policies in place, but also staff must be aware of their existence. A good time for this discussion is at a formally constructed and regularly carried-out introduction to an institution. By its very nature, missing documentation concerning human resource and staffing issues should arouse suspicion in those who are specifically seeking it. The inability to provide this information is an indicator of a negative culture.

Disciplinary procedures

There should be clear identification of a graded disciplinary process with counselling and personnel development at its core.

Staffing statistics

There must be evidence of regular review and documentation of staff turnover and sickness rates (both institutional and departmental), as well as up-to-date lists of staff who have resigned or who have been dismissed, with evidence of their exit interviews. Higher-than-expected staff turnover and sickness rates suggest unaddressed or unresolved problems, and they are often department- or division-specific. These are signs of a 'local negative culture' within an organization, and these features need to be reviewed on a regular basis by those responsible for HR activities. Any lack of these data is a sign of a negative culture and an insufficiently active HR department.

Staff satisfaction surveys

Although there are a number of commercial staff survey services available, they have in common both length and complexity. The purposes of staff surveys are twofold: first, to obtain information (recognizing that polling methods give biased results) and, second, to demonstrate that management is interested in the opinion and welfare of those who work in the organization. Consequently, 15–20 well-chosen questions on topics important to staff will help to identify those areas that need attention. Not all subjects can be studied simultaneously, but there are halo effects on the feeling of well-being of staff as the process evolves.

Policies and procedures

Total disclosure (transparency) policy

It is a common finding that, when an HR department or hospital administration is criticized, they close ranks and defend their positions. This is also a common response to patient complaints about the provision of healthcare or adjunct services. A declared and evident commitment to 'telling the truth' is necessary. Although it may seem strange to put this item in a list of requirements to identify a PMC, we believe that the majority of institutions declare honesty and transparency but function with concealment and protectionism. This is an area in which senior management must lead by example, because these principles are so easy to say but usually so difficult to fulfil. Those employed in intermediate and even quite senior management positions may believe that their first loyalty is to defend the institution against criticism. It requires senior leadership, by their example, to show how to undertake candid and open discussions in a friendly and objective fashion with those who are being critical in a hostile manner. The offer of an external objective review is often followed by a willingness to engage in a problem-solving exercise. In addition, there should be evidence that complaints and criticisms have been responded to with expediency. Delayed or protective responses are a sign of a 'negative culture'.

Performance management

The great majority of those in healthcare come to work on a daily basis setting out to do their best. For this majority, issues of performance improvement and counselling can be successfully achieved in an educational (formative) context. In contrast, for the minority who are unable to either recognize their deficiency or curb their disruptive behaviours, disciplinary (normative) procedures are needed and should be separate from and not mixed with educational remedial processes. The mixing of 'formative' and 'normative' performance improvement processes undermines the trust for educational endeavours to which the majority respond very positively and creates resistances from those who might otherwise be helped. Attempting to achieve performance improvement for the majority by using disciplinary methods is demotivating and counterproductive. Thus, we recommend that those involved with an institution's strategic organizational plan recognize the distinction between such 'formative' and 'normative' processes and use both separate structures and separate personnel for these activities.

Goals and objectives

Signs of a positive institutional cultural health include an organized approach to the identification of annual goals and objectives in the context of prestated vision and mission language, annual assessments against these goals and objectives (areas of achievement, partial achievement or no achievement), goals and objectives stated in specific language with measurable outcomes, and metrics of change and stated plans to either carry forward or abandon ideas as results are obtained. In addition, regularly produced and distributed newsletters (which can provide evidence of celebration of local achievements) are additional signs of a positive culture. The documentation of these functions should be available for the hospital in general and also for its subunits, along with departmental reports, minutes and attendance registers.

In contrast, features that are likely to be associated with broader negative culture include the documentation of institutional activity in reports written in broad and non-specific language. Sustained non-attendance for those groups/teams working on goals and objectives (which is most often observed with doctors) requires correction to prevent the practice of disruptive denial of project results and recommendations by those who practise chronic non-participation.

Performance indicators

Aggregate data at divisional and departmental levels are an essential prerequisite for an organized approach to clinical performance improvement. When no such data exists, it is likely that divisional or departmental reputation will be either defended by generalizations or protected by claims of confidentiality. If and when poor outcome data are identified, either from analysis of aggregate data or based on individual patient outcomes, the lack of an organized approach to data gathering and analysis may precipitate a negative cultural reaction for protectionism and self-serving denial. There must be a demonstration that performance information has been used to achieve change.[14]

Doctor variance

Although doctor-specific variance studies have been carried out for more than two decades[15-17] this sensitive subject engenders great reactivity by the medical profession in general and by the involved doctors in particular. In the context of addressing doctor-specific variance, there needs to be greater recognition of the value to distinguish between an educational approach (formative actions) in contrast to normative corrective/disciplinary actions in the resolution of these problems. However, the availability of 'score cards' and other forms of regular clinical governance reports containing individual results should be encouraged because it provides some degree of objectivity to the process. Minutes of regular peer review and audit meetings should be available, and attendance of members of the multidisciplinary teams (particularly of doctors) to support these activities is further evidence of a positive and forward-looking institutional culture.

A 'no-blame' environment

Although difficult to envision, critical incident reporting and review, peer review, and critical incident analysis should be constructed to achieve a 'no-blame' educational approach. Disciplinary remedy should be a separate process called upon when individuals or groups of individuals appear unable or unwilling to participate positively in the educational approach to problem remediation. Clearly stated, policies and procedures to accommodate a separate process to deal with situations of such 'disruption' should increase trust in educational processes. This will ensure that the majority of problem topics can and should be handled within the context of such a 'no-blame' educational environment in which systems rather than individuals are identified as giving rise to the error in the majority of cases.[18]

Process change and re-engineering

Although some processes in hospitals are complex, many are relatively simple or can be made so by re-engineering. There should be documented evidence in all parts of the hospital organization encouraging those working in these areas to make suggestions of process simplification and improvement. Along with this general philosophy of increased simplicity and diminished complexity should be a commitment to reducing the size of the hospital administration. There should be clearly defined organizational charts and plans in place to minimize administrative overhead. A consistent pattern of increased complexity, which is frequently associated with the creation of new administrative positions, may be a sign of poor morale and a negative cultural environment.

Reducing the complexity of systems and the redesigning of processes around the patient are among the basic tenets of clinical performance improvement. Some organizations are undertaking efforts in which redesign results in greater complexity, and these efforts seem counterproductive. If the process has been redesigned thoroughly, there will be no need for new administrative posts to monitor its implementation. Good design must include the routine capture of robust clinical information about both process and outcome. These data need not be complex, but should be reviewed regularly. Reports by exception are a useful approach.

Risk management

Records concerning critical incident reviews conducted in a non-judgmental fashion with neutral identification of facts, root-cause analysis, as well as process and personnel errors, require considerable administrative skill to prevent 'finger pointing' and blame attribution. The format for these discussions to support a positive culture should be that all concerned meet together, preferably with a facilitator dedicated to the precepts of a positive cultural environment.

For those who have the responsibility of assessing this aspect of institutional culture, confidential questioning of those who have been involved in recent clinical incident reviews should use words and statements so that the individuals feel supported by the process. In contrast, staff members who are reticent to be truthful and fear retribution and negative repercussions are signs that cultural improvement is needed.

The appropriate management of clinical risk is fundamental to the clinical governance process. Properly concluded multidisciplinary critical incident reviews can only be carried out if there are designated trained staff from a *different department* prepared to lead this process and determine root causes. In addition, if the information is not collected in an independent fashion, trend analyses will not be possible and lessons learnt will be lost. There should be well-maintained risk-management databases with evidence of critical incident reviews with remedial action plans that have been monitored and implemented. There should also be evidence that incident reports made by staff members from all areas of the institution have been addressed and resolved in a reasonable timeframe. Staff who have reported these incidents should be made aware that their concerns have been addressed. However, confidential remediation plans and actions should not be divulged, because of confidentiality issues. Complainants usually find that not knowing the specifics of an outcome is frustrating, but those who are in remediation also have rights of privacy. Therefore, individual staff should be made aware that incident reports have resulted in changed processes or procedures. This type of post-incident awareness is a sign of a positive culture.

Environmental issues

The general appearance of a facility may be helpful in identifying an institution with high morale and a positive culture. Clean institutional appearance, empty litter bins, removal of clinical and non-clinical waste, removal of wilting flowers and other debris, and lack of graffiti in public areas, elevators, staircases and toilets all attest to the creation of a positive environment and culture. These are signs that staff take pride in and are engaged with the institution.

Customer service

Wayfinding

Bright and well-posted signs in an institution, as well as helpful staff, are always reassuring to patients as they navigate their way to or from a particular area. Staff members all being prepared to offer assistance when members of the public appear lost or distressed is also consistent with a broader positive environment.

Concurrent information

There are opportunities during the intermissions between the activities of healthcare provision when we can seek the opinions of patients concerning their needs and whether we have met their expectations. Very simple questions such as 'Is there anything more I can do to help?', 'Are you warm enough?', 'Do you understand what is happening at the moment?' can generate the sense that we are being patient-centred in our approach. The need for this form of interaction on a regular and routine basis should be covered in the orientation process for new staff and also demonstrated by senior management as they walk around.

Retrospective surveys

Simply constructed short surveys concerning the hotel functions and general well-being of patients are usually illuminating, particularly when simple Likert (1–5) scales are used and the results aggregated. Action taken on those areas of suboptimal performance is further evidence of a positive and outward-looking institutional culture.

Discussion

Implementation of the cultural changes needed to achieve the prerequisites of clinical governance requires a major shift in attitude, which must be achieved by a broad spectrum of healthcare staff at all levels. This transition[19] is both an administrative and a psychological process, the pace of which cannot be forced. If change is seen to be imposed, additional problems are created for those who have the responsibility to achieve the desired result.

> 'There is nothing more difficult to carry out, nor more doubtful of success, nor more dangerous to handle than to initiate a new order of things. For the reformer has enemies in all who profit by the old order and only lukewarm defenders in those who would profit by the new order.'
>
> Machiavelli (1513)

Central government has not always helped to achieve a focus on performance improvement, because a plethora of new targets have been identified, in addition to the creation of directives and inspectorates.[20-23] These actions have created a climate of mistrust and confusion that does not easily lend itself to the developments described in this chapter aimed at PMC improvement.

To cope and deliver on an agenda of modernization and reform, there must be both central and local leaderships clearly devoted to two constituents: first, the population that they serve, and, second, the staff who do the work. The mechanical view that 'healthcare workers' are merely cogs in the machine to be directed and driven must give way to a more nurturing approach of respect, support and accountability, emerging as the model for new and more productive healthcare.[24-27] We believe that the cultural indicators summarized in this chapter can be used to clearly identify those organizations that are better able to support and maintain a continuous quality improvement programme. In contrast, it should be possible, by using these indicators, to identify those organizations in which unacceptable practices and less than adequate clinical outcomes can occur without the accountability being demanded by society.

It is clear that the cultural indicators described here are not an exhaustive list of those features that can be identified within a positive healthcare delivery approach. Rather, this chapter should be seen as a starting point for those who have responsibility for institutional development and those who have the task to assess their progress.

Acknowledgements

We gratefully acknowledge the advice provided to us by Nancy Dixon, Sue Shultz and Mary Chambers in the preparation of this chapter.

References

1. Mead M (ed). *Cultural Patterns and Technical Change.* UNESCO, 1953.
2. Ham C, Alberti KG. The medical profession, the public, and the government. *BMJ* 2002; **324:** 838–42.
3. Institute of Medicine. *To Err is Human: Building a Safer Health System.* National Academies Press, 2000.
4. Institute of Medicine, Committee on Quality of Healthcare in America. *Crossing the Quality Chasm: A New Health System for the 21st Century.* National Academies Press, 2001.
5. *Learning from Bristol: The Report Of The Public Inquiry Into Children's Heart Surgery At The Bristol Royal Infirmary 1984–1995.* London: HMSO, 2001 (http://www.doh.gov.uk/bristolinquiryresponse).
6. Day P, Klein R. Who nose best? Commission for Health Improvement. *Health Serv J* 2002; **112:** 26–9.
7. Center for the Evaluation of Clinical Sciences Staff. *The Dartmouth Atlas of Health Care.* American Hospital Assocation, 1999.
8. www.doh.gov.uk/performanceindicators/2002.
9. Maxwell RJ Dimensions of quality revisited: from thought to action. *Qual Health Care* 1992, **1:** 171–7.
10. Davies HT, Nutley SM, Mannion R. Organisational culture and quality of healthcare. *Qual Health Care* 2000; **9:** 111–19.
11. Shortell SM, Bennett CL, Byck GR. Assessing the impact of continuous quality improvement on clinical practice; what it will take to accelerate progress. *Milbank Q* 1998; **76:** 593–624, 510.

12. Fielding LP. Clinical governance: The conflicts within performance improvement. Modernising the NHS – Delivering Quality in a Complex Environment. Forum on Quality in Healthcare at the Royal Society of Medicine, London, 7 November 2001.

13. Goleman D. *Emotional Intelligence*. New York: Bantam Books, 1995.

14. Hittinger R. Using clinical performance indicators to achieve clinical governance. *Clin Governance Bull* 2002; **3:** 4–5, (http://www.rsm.ac.uk/pub/cbgmay02.pdf).

15. Fielding LP, Stewart-Brown S, Dudley HA. Surgeon related variables and the clinical trial. *Lancet* 1978; **ii:** 778–9.

16. Phillips RKS, Hittinger R, Blesovsky L *et al.* Local recurrence after curative surgery for large bowel cancer: I. The overall picture. *Br J Surg* 1984; **71:** 12–16.

17. Phillips RKS, Hittinger R, Blesovsky L *et al.* Local recurrence after curative surgery for large bowel cancer: II. The rectum and rectosigmoid. *Br J Surg* 1984; **71:** 17–20.

18. Reason J. Human error: models and management. *BMJ* 2000; **320:** 768–70.

19. Bridges W. *Managing Transitions*. Boston: Addison-Wesley, 1991.

20. Walshe K. The rise of regulation in the NHS. *BMJ* 2002; **324:** 967–70.

21. Dewar S, Findlayson B. The I in the new CHAI. *BMJ* 2002; **325:** 848–50.

22. Burde H. The implementation of quality and safety measures: from rhetoric to reality. *J Health Law* 2002; **35:** 263–81.

23. Managed care: a rationing-by-deterrence mechanism that doesn't reduce quality of care (?). In: Shenkin HA (ed). *Myths in Medical Care: Causes and Effects*. Danbury, CT: Rutledge Books, 2000: 103–21.

24. Plsek PE, Greenhalgh T. Complexity science: The challenge of complexity in health care. *BMJ* 2001; **323:** 625–8.

25. Wilson T, Holt T. Complexity science: complexity and clinical care. *BMJ* 2001; **323:** 685–8.

26. Plsek PE, Wilson T. Complexity, leadership, and management in healthcare organisations. *BMJ* 2001; **323:** 746–9.

27. Fraser SW, Greenhalgh T. Coping with complexity: educating the capability. *BMJ* 2001; **323:** 799–803.

4

Care pathways: Improving the patient journey

Siân Jones

'It is good to have an end to journey towards, but it is the journey that matters, in the end.'

Ursula K LeGuin

Background

A journey involves travel across varied terrain, encountering different people, potential delays and a range of information from different sources – there may also be more than one way of reaching the destination. The series of experiences that a patient or user of healthcare services encounters can be compared to a journey. What makes a good journey is the quality of the experience.

The steps involved in an episode of care often involve a range of staff and departments and encompass numerous processes, both within and outside the hospital setting. These steps are usually dependent on memory and routine, which can be easily influenced by factors such as medical staff turnover and bank or agency staff who may not be familiar with the processes involved. The progression of the patient journey across departments and into different sectors increases the possibility of communication breakdown, resulting in duplication or omission of steps in the process.

The clinical governance framework requires the application of systems in order to promote quality; clinicians do not always have the time available to develop these systems. Some kind of 'tool' is therefore needed to encompass elements of routine practice, to form a structured means of implementing the best evidence, to improve standards of care.[1] As a tool for clinical governance (Figure 4.1), care pathways form an approach to patient care that meets these requirements, including continuous evaluation, evidence-based practice, joint-working, clinical audit and the patient experience.[2]

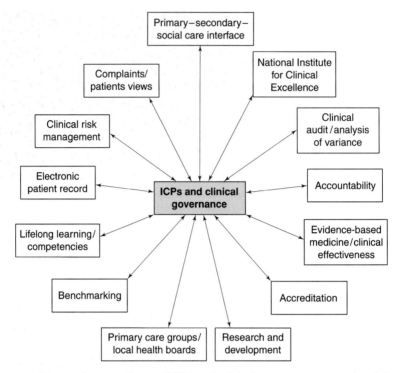

FIGURE 4.1 Integrated care pathways (ICPs) and clinical governance. Reproduced from the 'What is …' series by kind permission of Hayward Medical Communications.

Originating in the USA, where they were developed to ensure high-quality care, while controlling costs, care pathways are now being used widely across the UK in a range of settings. At the time of their introduction in the late 1980s, further emphasis was placed on the importance of evidence-based medicine and close examination of clinical practice in the NHS, alongside cost effectiveness and efficiency.[3] With greater reference to care pathways in initiatives such as National Service Frameworks and by the Healthcare Commission, the adoption of this tool to improve healthcare delivery has become more widespread. With the further development of health technology, reference has also been made to care pathways in the NHS information strategy *Delivering 21st Century IT for the NHS*;[4] this identifies electronic care pathways (eICPs) as a significant contributor to the evaluation of healthcare. There are now web-based discussion sites, regional user-groups, conferences and training opportunities all dedicated to care pathways; the National Electronic Library for Health (NeLH) maintains a database of examples of care pathways.[5]

The benefits of care pathways have been shown to be widespread. For the patient, they provide an opportunity for greater involvement in care,[6] enhanced communication with health professionals and increased satisfaction.[7] The emphasis made by care pathways on multiprofessional working promotes a clearer understanding of roles for clinical staff and improved communication; time spent on documentation is reduced[8] and seamless care is promoted across all boundaries. In addition, care pathways are an effective means of evaluating and making better use of resources, identifying 'bottlenecks' in services and reducing duplication and, potentially, costs by the streamlining of processes.

What is meant by a care pathway?

With the increasing prevalence of care pathways in both the NHS and private health sector, more health professionals are becoming familiar with the term 'care pathway'. Although awareness is improving, there is still some ambiguity over what constitutes a 'care pathway'. Prior to the introduction of a framework for care pathway development at Cardiff and Vale NHS Trust, a baseline review identified 46 'care pathways'. Of these, 25 consisted of several algorithms, an assessment tool, procedural checklists and a nursing care plan, as well as some examples of integrated notes for specific episodes of care. This varied application of the term 'care pathway' appears to be common.[9] The care pathway tool is distinct from flowchart 'pathways',[10] although the flowchart (or algorithm) is a useful part of the process in outlining a visual representation of the patient journey.

A definition helps to promote clarity. One definition, devised by the National Pathways Association[11] and frequently referred to, summarizes some of the key features:

> 'An integrated care pathway determines locally agreed multidisciplinary practice based on guidelines and evidence where available for a specific patient/client group. It forms all or part of the clinical record, documents the care given and facilitates the evaluation of outcomes for continuous quality improvement.'

A care pathway outlines a plan of care within a defined timeframe; it involves a process of review of current practice and the streamlining of documentation to create a single, multiprofessional record of care: the care pathway tool. Several factors that stem from a changing NHS environment, such as empowerment of patients, clinical governance and the proposed development of electronic patient records, indicate a need for structured documentation, such as that provided by care pathways.

What makes the care pathway tool unique is the incorporation of a means for monitoring anticipated care against actual care through the recording of 'variances'. This built-in audit mechanism allows for flexibility in the use of the care pathway tool, ensuring that it not only meets the individual needs of patients, but also recognizes the issue of clinical freedom in decision making by clinicians. The care pathway tool forms a framework for best practice; it is not prescriptive, but acts as a guide to clinical staff and allows for variability in practice. This variability is recorded within an appropriate section of the care pathway tool as a 'variance'; anything that takes place in relation to the patient's management that is not identified by the care pathway tool is a variance. This will be expanded upon in a later section.

Developing a care pathway

'To make improvements, we must be clear about what we are trying to accomplish, how we will know that a change has led to improvement and what change we can make that will result in improvement.'

Dr Don Berwick, President/CEO, Institute of Healthcare Improvement

The process of care pathway development requires clarification from the beginning of desired outcomes and a means of evaluation, to ensure that the time and energy invested by all involved makes a difference to care delivery. Care pathway development can:

- reduce variation in practice
- improve communication with patients/users
- implement guidelines into practice
- reduce inconsistent practice
- address complaints
- reduce fragmentation of care
- improve multiprofessional team coordination

Developing a care pathway involves a process of change; the identification of clinical 'champions' to support and drive the work is one of the key factors that promotes success of this process. A development group made up of committed representatives of all the professions involved is established; patient input is also required to ensure that the care pathway is designed to accommodate their perspective. Involvement of the patient viewpoint in care pathway development allows:

- involvement of patient representatives in the development group
- the use of information gained from focus group activity
- the use of complaints data
- patient satisfaction surveys

The involvement of care pathways in service delivery can be seen as a means of redesigning processes of treatment and care. Achieving this involves consideration of whether the right people are doing the right thing, at the right time, and in the right place.

Being more specific about the above has been identified as one means of improving guideline implementation.[12] The difficulty in encouraging the use of guidelines in practice has been recognized;[13] the care pathway tool promotes the use of guidelines 'at the bedside'. The format encourages clarification of role and activities.

The process of developing a care pathway involves review of existing practice and consensus within the team regarding the way forward, to ensure improvement. This improvement is based on the need for clinical practice to be evidence-based (where possible) and streamlined: any duplication is identified and roles are clarified. This is also a good opportunity to review patient information and the clinical documentation of all professional groups. The quality and usefulness of current clinical record keeping has been recognized;[14] the development of a care pathway provides an ideal opportunity for a structure to be incorporated that encourages more accurate recording of information. Documentation is streamlined and incorporated into a single multiprofessional record for the use of all staff; this replaces existing uniprofessional record keeping. Documentation becomes the care pathway tool – the framework that supports the clinical team in the implementation of consistent, quality care. Professional guidelines for record keeping should be referred to when formatting the care pathway; the development of a template using this information can be helpful to staff.

At Cardiff and Vale NHS Trust, a model has been established for the development of care pathways, to promote a consistent approach (Figure 4.2); a full-time care pathways manager and administrative assistant are available to help coordinate the individual care pathway projects, providing information, guidance and support in documentation design. At Cardiff, each care pathway project must be identified as a priority for the particular directorate and incorporated into the rolling audit programme. By doing this, care pathways become part of the routine practice of service improvement.

The expansion in the use of information technology and evolution of the electronic patient record will greatly enhance the way in which care pathways are developed and used in the future: wider access to information as IT hardware becomes more readily available; electronic completion of the care pathway and, as a result, direct collection of variance data; improved access to the care pathway, by more than one person at a time; and tighter version control.

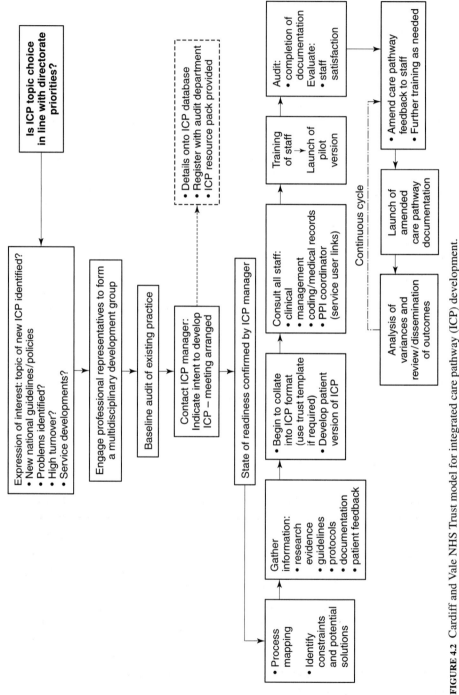

FIGURE 4.2 Cardiff and Vale NHS Trust model for integrated care pathway (ICP) development.

Variances: adding flexibility

A care pathway is a dynamic tool that requires frequent review and updating, through the monitoring of variances, to ensure that it continues to meet the needs of the patient group and that it remains a source of best practice. Variances are the built-in audit mechanism that allow for comparison to be made between the *anticipated* plan of care and what *actually* happens.

Variances contribute to the flexibility of a care pathway tool. Pareto's principle can be applied here, to illustrate that the care pathway will meet the needs of 80% of the specified patient population and the remaining 20% will show some degree of variance. Recognizing these variances and acting upon them allows the care pathway to be flexible. Variances may occur in relation to the individual needs of the patient, or as a response to a particular intervention; they may be categorized as relating to the patient, staff, system (i.e. healthcare processes/systems), or social (i.e. home circumstances). Variances also allow for healthcare professionals to exercise their own professional judgement, as long as any alteration in practice is recorded as a variance and can be justified. The care pathway design includes a section for the recording of variances that should ideally be situated adjacent to the account of clinical interventions/activities (Table 4.1).

This mechanism for flexibility in the care pathway tool should be emphasized when introducing it to a member of staff for the first time; care pathways are criticized due to the general misunderstanding that they are prescriptive protocols, unable to take individual patient need or professional judgement into account.

Ownership

From the beginning of the process, it is important to ensure that the wider team is aware of the work taking place around the development of the care pathway. This promotes a sense of ownership and involvement, which will contribute to the success of the care pathway. It can be done through briefings at, for example, existing ward meetings, away-days and clinical governance sessions, and by the use of notice boards in clinical areas. Once a draft of the documentation (the care pathway tool) has been developed, it is useful to get feedback from staff regarding how user-friendly it appears to be; these comments are then incorporated (where appropriate) into the design, prior to the pilot phase. The true test of the care pathway tool will be its use in the clinical setting – too much time is often spent fine-tuning the content and layout prior to its practical application, which is often an unnecessary waste of resources.

TABLE 4.1 Example of variance recording

(i) This table is an example of a section of a page from a care pathway tool, based on the Cardiff and Vale NHS Trust template. Pages such as this are set out across the specified timeframe (e.g. days, hours, stages), outlining clinical activities and interventions based on best practice. Where an activity is not carried out, the 'unmet' column is marked with a cross and details are recorded in the accompanying variance section (ii).

Clinical activity	Met ☑	Unmet ☒ (Variance: record in variance table)	Signature
1.0 Assessment			
1.1 Reviewed by medical staff	☑	☐	*P Thomas*
1.2 Observations of HR, BP, temp, SaO$_2$ recorded 4-hourly by nurse	☑	☐	*S Evans*
1.3 Blood loss monitored at drain site	☑	☐	*S Evans*
2.0 Medication			
2.1 Pain monitored and PCA discontinued when pain controlled	☑	☐	*S Evans*
2.2 Discontinue IVI if patient tolerating fluids	☑	☐	*S Evans*
3.0 Mobility			
3.1 Commence gentle mobilizing around bed area	☐	☒	*S Evans*
3.2 Ensure anti-embolus stockings correctly *in situ*	☑	☐	*S Evans*

(ii) The variance information recorded here refers to clinical activity code 3.1, under 'Mobility' in (i). Reviewing this information provides a valuable insight into how comparable actual care is to that outlined by the care pathway's best practice framework.

Time	Clinical activity code	Variance	Reason for variance	Action taken	Signature
09 15	3.1	Unable to mobilize	Nausea and vomiting	IM Stemetil given, 12.5 mg	*S Evans*

The team developing the care pathway should ensure that it is amended as necessary to accommodate any new guidelines or evidence. This ongoing review process keeps the care pathway 'alive' whilst ensuring continuous quality improvement.

CASE STUDY 1 – where limited involvement leads to poor use of the care pathway tool

A strong top–down drive for change and improvement in thrombolysis administration times promoted the development of a care pathway for myocardial infarction within a tight timeframe; this timeframe also happened to include the Christmas period! A version of the care pathway from a neighbouring trust was adapted for local use. Despite being aware of the need to consult with representatives of the wider clinical team involved in the episode of care, only the care pathway coordinator and one consultant worked on the development of the care pathway tool, with separate input from a senior nurse. Time pressures did not allow for a more rigorous approach to be taken, as outlined in care pathway texts. The clinical demands during this busy winter period and the absence of staff due to Christmas meant that any form of awareness and training was very limited. As a result, the launch in the new year of the care pathway in the clinical area was met with confusion, cynicism and disinterest; some staff did try to use it, but their unfamiliarity with the documentation meant that their attempts were often futile. A staff survey indicated that they did not understand why it had been introduced, whether it was to be used in addition to conventional documentation and who should complete which section; one of the professional groups felt that it did not fully represent their aspects of care and that there were some serious omissions. A new version was devised soon after, with local involvement, resulting in greater satisfaction.

Lessons learnt

- Clinical policy demands often make it difficult to follow the ideal process for developing a care pathway; frequently, a degree of flexibility and pragmatism is required during the process, which may still achieve the desired outcomes. However, the greater the digression from the ideal, the lower the chance of success.
- Input in the development process of the care pathway is crucial to ensuring that all staff users of the care pathway tool are aware of its purpose and understand how it can be used.
- As the care pathway tool is an evolving, dynamic means of improving healthcare delivery, some mistakes can be afforded during the development and implementation of the first version; when a team is new to care pathways, this is often inevitable. However, lack of involvement of those who will be using the care pathway can result in anti care pathway sentiment; it is fortunate that the example outlined here resulted in the interest of staff to persevere and accept further developments to the care pathway. This is likely to have been due to good support and leadership from senior members of the team.

The patient version

A patient/user version of the care pathway tool is an effective means of involving individuals in their own care, as well as providing information. This may consist of a summary sheet, outlining key activities and interventions, along the timeframe of a particular episode of care (Table 4.2). Although there is often concern that complaints and dissatisfaction will increase should any of these events not occur when expected, care pathways have been shown to reduce complaints and incidences of litigation.[15]

The patient version of the care pathway tool is provided at the start of the episode of care as one means of providing information; it complements patient information booklets/leaflets and verbal information. The care pathway process provides a good opportunity to review existing patient information to determine whether it is of good quality and up-to-date.

Making it work

> 'All improvement requires change and improving quality in healthcare involves changing the way that things are done, change in processes and in the behaviour of people and teams of people.'[16]

Although there is now more guidance available on how to develop care pathways, putting this into practice is not always as straightforward as it may seem. The introduction of any new way of working stimulates a range of responses according to whether the stakeholders view it as a threat or an opportunity. Care pathways come with their own baggage of myths and legends; a 'Chinese whispers' effect across areas that have no experience of developing care pathways does little to support their introduction. Medical staff refer to the 'cookbook' nature of the care pathway tool[17] and the threat that this poses to their autonomy. 'Initiative fatigue' reduces the interest in care pathways, which may be perceived as 'just the latest thing' among a series of management techniques that appear to readily come and go. In addition, care pathways are often considered to be nursing initiatives, elaborate care plans that have no place for medical involvement.

The process of change

The development of a care pathway stimulates change. It allows clinicians to re-evaluate services, to ensure the best possible outcome for patients, and to ensure that care is evidence-based, of good quality, cost-effective and efficient.

TABLE 4.2 Patient version (postoperative episode)

	Day of surgery	Day 1	Day 2	Day of discharge
Visits to ward from healthcare staff	The surgeon will visit you	The doctors will see you	The doctors will see you	The doctors will see you
Tests	—	You will have blood tests.	—	—
Observations	Observations of your pulse and blood pressure will be taken frequently. The wound will be checked. Your temperature will also be recorded	The observations will only be recorded every 4 hours. The wound will be checked	The observations will only be recorded every 4 hours	The observations will only be recorded every 4 hours, until you go home
Medication/treatments	Nurses will monitor your pain, and medication will be given to you as required. You will have a catheter in your bladder. There will be a drip in your arm	The nurse will monitor your pain, and you will be given medication for this	The catheter will be removed. The drip will be taken out of your arm	You will be given tablets to take home
Eating/drinking	Sips of fluid, increasing to frequent drinks	Eat normally. Have frequent drinks; the nurses will monitor this with you	Eat normally	Eat normally
Hygiene	Nurses will help you to have a wash	You may have a shower. The nurse may help you if necessary	You may shower independently	You may shower independently
Activity	You will stay in bed supported by pillows	Walk around gradually for short periods, with assistance	Increased episodes of walking	Continue to increase time and lengths of walks
Information	The surgeon and the nurses will be happy to discuss any concerns you may have	The ward staff will be happy to discuss any concerns you may have	The ward staff will be happy to discuss any concerns you may have	You will be given an information booklet by the ward staff

In order to do this, all professions involved are required to come together, to share information, perceptions and experiences, and to appreciate each others' roles and viewpoint on the service. This change can potentially create tension between the balance of the existing power structure between the professional groups involved. As an agent for change,[7] a care pathway generates new ways of working, closer multiprofessional liaison and the integration of clinical notes; in addition, the use of the care pathway tool itself, at the bedside, brings guidelines 'to life' as they are built into the care pathway format and used directly with the patient.

At Cardiff and Vale, the care pathway process was initiated across the Trust by identifying areas of interest and enthusiasm. Champions – key, supportive stakeholders – were identified in these areas; this type of individual has been recognized as a means of ensuring that the change process is successful.[18] At Cardiff, medical champions were found to be of most benefit in leading the projects and involving and persuading junior doctors to become involved. The identification of champions to support the change process was complemented by a care pathways awareness programme, which included a multiprofessional conference.[19]

Critical success factors

Medical involvement

As previously indicated, medical involvement is one of the crucial success factors in care pathway development.[20] Resistance to care pathways is frequently strongest among medical staff, mainly due to the structured format of the tool itself. Despite awareness of this and the involvement of senior medical champions, there are still incidences at Cardiff and elsewhere[21] where junior doctors' compliance is a problem. This is not improved by their frequent changeover periods. In some cases, the involvement of nurse practitioners has improved the situation: for example, in the Emergency Unit, where care pathways are providing supportive, evidence-based frameworks for emergency nurse practitioners (ENPs) to manage the care of self-poisoning cases. These nurses are permanent members of staff with wide experience and knowledge; the care pathways have been devised with the involvement of medical staff to give them supportive framework to develop extended roles.

Facilitation

The significant value of facilitation in the development of care pathways has been recognized;[8,17] this view is reflected by the experience at Cardiff and Vale.

CASE STUDY 2 – encouraging use of the care pathway tool by doctors

Experience from the development of an emergency medical admissions assessment tool at Cardiff and Vale NHS Trust indicated that medical staff did not like the structured layout of the medical clerking section, preferring blank sections to record details of their assessment and examination. The purpose of this tool was to reduce variation in the recording of information and improve communication across the Emergency Department and wards areas. It was already understood that medical staff found the format of care pathways too structured and even prescriptive. As a result, the first step in the development of many of the care pathway tools has been the creation of an integrated clinical record, ensuring that all professional groups, including doctors, are contributing to this *only* and not their own professional records. A limited amount of the standard care pathway format is included in the medical sections of each stage of the care pathway, such as a few key prompts and space to record any variances from the expected practice, but much of the rest remains as free text space. The structure of care pathways promotes a more consistent approach while building guidelines into practice; the other professional groups are more suited to this format, as it fits in with the way they work, using proformas, care plans and assessments.

Lessons learnt

- This approach has improved compliance by doctors with many of the care pathways.
- Feedback from the use of this first version identifies where some additional structure could potentially produce better results, steering the design more towards that of a decision support framework.
- The new way of working introduced by care pathways is a difficult change for most healthcare staff; during busy periods new documentation that is unfamiliar and non-user-friendly is likely to be disregarded. Although it takes time, the gradual step-by-step development of the care pathway tool, including feedback as each version is implemented, is more likely to be accepted.

Prior to the appointment of a full-time facilitator, several care pathway projects had been initiated but had stalled due to other commitments of those involved and poor project management; one example had been in progress for two years, without reaching a pilot phase. Care pathway development is frequently an add-on to existing clinical commitments, and consequently keeping to timeframes and maintaining motivation can be difficult. The facilitator does not have to be from a clinical background, but could for example have audit experience or have worked in project management; their role is to train staff, increase awareness and project-manage the work.

Information technology

As long as care pathways exist in a paper format, there will be difficulties linked to the lack of comprehensive information systems. The built-in audit mechanism provided by variances generates important data, which requires systems to ensure that it is collected and analysed. Access to IT hardware, such as a computer, can be limited in clinical areas, which rules out the use of electronic completion of the care pathway tool. The future arrangements proposed through national IM&T strategy should resolve some of these difficulties, but in the meantime the process of evaluation is done retrospectively and laboriously. At Cardiff and Vale, informal surveys in parts of the trust have identified computers that are inaccessible out of hours due to their location in administrative offices; providing limited and controlled access to those that are near to the clinical areas allows staff to format care pathway documentation themselves and access literature databases via the NHS Wales intranet.

Leadership

Any process of change requires good leadership, to steer the activity, maintain a focus on the objectives and motivate the team. For a wide programme of care pathways to be successful, it must have the backing of the organization, including visible commitment from senior management. Each individual care pathway team must identify a lead clinician to drive the work; this is usually a medical consultant. The experience at Cardiff and Vale shows that those care pathways with an identified supportive and committed consultant as the project lead have a greater success rate.

Breaking the journey into chunks

Care pathways often fail when those involved in the development have been over-ambitious in its scope (i.e. the span of the pathway between the start and end of a specified episode of care). The overall journey can be mapped out by the development team, but it is often easier and more successful to break it down into smaller chunks when designing the care pathway. Each of these chunks can then flow into the others as they are developed. For example, for a patient with a stroke:

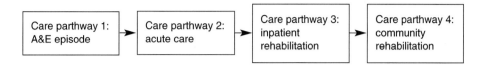

Each of these forms a single care pathway, linking into each other to outline the patient journey. In developing smaller sections, the process is quicker; it is also good for those who are new to the process. Individual care pathway chunks may remain within a single sector or may cross boundaries, depending on where the start and end points are set.

A better patient journey

> 'The traveller has reached the end of the journey!'
> Edmund Burke

Once at their destination, the individual may look back and reflect on the experience of the journey; a good, safe experience of high quality is often created through careful planning and process design. It is the same with a care pathway: the importance of the process of development cannot be stressed enough. Often the focus is on the documentation – the care pathway tool – but without adequate attention to the steps of development, the effectiveness of the care pathway will be limited.[17] A well-designed care pathway that takes into consideration the issues previously outlined has good potential for improving the patient journey.

As a patient-centred approach, care pathways are a useful means of increasing patient involvement in the planning of healthcare processes.[17] The involvement of patients, service users and carers is increasingly being encouraged and recognized as a valuable means of understanding their viewpoint of healthcare; this input informs the development of services that are designed much more around the user than the organization or its staff. In relation to the development of clinical guidelines, the Scottish Intercollegiate Guidelines Network (SIGN) suggest the following:

> Patients and carers may have different perspectives on healthcare processes, priorities and outcomes from those of health professionals. The involvement of patients, carers or their representatives in guideline development is therefore important to help ensure that guidelines reflect their needs and concerns.

This same principle can be applied to the development of care pathways. As indicated above, there does need to be some structure to the care pathway development process, but, in order for aspects of care that are important to the patient to be considered and converted to quality measures, there should be a degree of flexibility in the process and good levels of communication between healthcare professionals and patients.[22]

The National Patient Safety Agency[23] claims that the patient experience is at the centre of their aim to improve patient safety. The care pathway provides a suitable framework to support a safe journey for patients. The clarification of existing roles and development of new ones, based on appropriate skills and competencies, can make a difference to the patient experience and is part of the care pathway process; the NHS Modernisation Agency's *10 High Impact Changes*[24] identifies the redesign and extension of roles as a significant means of making a difference to key areas and emphasizes the effect that this can have on reducing errors and mistakes and improving patient care.

In addition, the development of a care pathway is a suitable opportunity to review issues around risk management; this can be a powerful means of identifying where potential for risk may occur, or responding to existing examples of clinical risk. The structure of care pathways in the Accident and Emergency Department at Cardiff has supported the extension of nurses' roles, to ensure that boundaries are clearly set as ENPs take on more of what was previously the doctors' responsibility; this has also been demonstrated in other organizations.[25]

In developing a care pathway, the impact on the journey should be to ensure that there is a consistent route to reach the destination, that this route is appropriately followed by all involved and is based on the best practice guidance available, that it involves value time for the patient, wherever possible, and that the information provided is timely and of good quality. The evaluation of the care pathway, through audit of variances, ensures that, where it is not suited to the specific patient population it is designed for, it can be adjusted; this 'live' feature of the care pathway tool ensures that it can continuously respond to incidents such as those relating to complaints or clinical risk.

Conclusion

The integrated care pathway provides a commonsense means of incorporating elements of clinical governance into routine care; this tool formalizes existing processes under one umbrella, promoting more effective and higher-quality practice. With patients contributing to the process, there is good scope for ensuring that the journey is tailored more specifically to their needs, increasing its value and improving the experience.

References

1. Johnson S. It ain't what you do, it's the way that you do it. *J Integrated Care Pathways* 2001; **5**: 26–8.
2. Bender AD, Motley RJ, Pierotti RJ *et al*. Quality and outcome management in primary care practice. *J Med Pract Manage* 1999; **14**: 236–40.
3. Middleton S, Roberts A. *Clinical Pathways Workbook*. The Health Quality Service, in association with The Kings Fund, 1998.
4. *Delivering 21st Century IT Support for the NHS: National Strategic Programme*. London: Department of Health, 2002.
5. Care Pathway Library, National Electronic Library for Health: http://libraries.nelh.nhs.uk/pathways/.
6. Williams JG, Roberts R, Rigby MJ. Integrated patient records: another move towards quality for patients? *Qual Health Care* 1993; **2**: 73–4.
7. De Luc K. Care pathways: an evaluation of their effectiveness. *J Adv Nurs* 2000; **32**: 485–96.
8. Johnson S, Smith J. Factors influencing the success of ICP projects. *Prof Nurse* 2000; **12**: 776–9.
9. Poole P, Johnson S. Integrated care pathways: an orthopaedic experience. *Physiotherapy* 1996; **82**: 28–30.
10. Johnson S, Dracass M, Vartan J *et al*. Setting standards using integrated care pathways. *Prof Nurse* 2000; **15**: 640–3.
11. Riley K. *National Pathways Association Newsletter* 1998; Spring: 2.
12. Michie S, Johnston M. Changing clinical behaviour by making guidelines specific. *BMJ* 2004; **328**: 343–5.
13. Grimshaw JM, Shirran L, Thomas R *et al*. Changing provider behaviour: an overview of systematic reviews of interventions. *Med Care* 2001; **39**(Suppl 2): 2–45.
14. Gabbay J, Layton AJ. Evaluation of audit of medical inpatient records in a district general hospital. *Qual Health Care* 1993; **1**: 43–7.
15. De Luc K. Are different models of care pathways being developed? *Int J Healthcare Qual Assur* 2000; **13**: 80–6.
16. Garside P. Organisational context for quality: lessons from the fields of organisational development and change management. *Qual HealthCare* 1998; **7** (Suppl): S8–15 (www.bmj.com/misc/qhc/30–36.shtml).
17. De Luc K. *Developing Care Pathways*. Oxford: Radcliffe Medical Press, 2001.
18. Hayes J. *The Theory and Practice of Change Management*. New York: Palgrave, 2002:106–7.
19. Jones SE. Spreading the word – one organisation's experience of holding an integrated care pathway awareness event. *J Integrated Care Pathways* 2004; **8**: 44–7.
20. Johnson S. The development and implementation of pathways in an acute setting. In: Wilson J (ed). *Integrated Care Management: The Path to Success?* Oxford: Butterworth-Heinemann, 1997:36–51.
21. CRAG Scottish Care Pathway Report: http://www.icpus.ukprofessionals.com/CRAGICPSummary.doc.
22. Smith E, Ross F. *Patient Experiences of Care Pathways: Cataract, Hip Replacement and Knee Arthroscopy – A Review of the Literature for the Commission for Health Improvement*. Nursing Research Unit, Kings College London, March 2004.
23. National Patient Safety Agency: http://www.npsa.nhs.uk/

24. Change number 10: redesign and extend roles in line with efficient patient pathways to attract and retain an efficient workforce. In: *10 High Impact Changes*. London: NHS Modernisation Agency, 2004.

25. Layton A, Moss F, Morgan G. Mapping out the patient's journey: experiences of developing pathways of care. *Qual Health Care* 1998; **7**(Suppl); S30–6 (www.bmj.com/misc/qhc/30–36.shtml).

5

Back to the future: Infection control moves back to the heart of corporate governance

Louise Teare

When hospitals were small and matron ruled, infection control was part of the corporate governance of the time. As hospitals have become more complex, procedures more invasive and public expectation greater, the potential for healthcare-associated infection (HCAI) has risen sharply. This has been confounded by the enormous amount of antibiotics used and the increasing resistance in association with the microbial 'struggle for survival'.

Healthcare presents a risk of infection

Exposure to any kind of healthcare presents a risk of infection. Recent government initiatives have recognized the importance of this and the need for infection control to be embedded within corporate governance of organizations.[1-4]

Trusts are increasingly using the balanced score card approach as the foundation for both strategic planning and operational delivery of services, identifying a comprehensive balance between parameters chosen (Figure 5.1). The new approach to infection control requires that Trusts must develop systems that allow infection control to enter and be part of this balanced score card.

Over the years, in spite of enormous strides by infection control teams, corporate management has tended to delegate infection control responsibility and has not itself been made accountable for developing adequate systems to control the risk of infection. Infection control teams have done their best, but often with inadequate resources and insufficient empowerment to make a difference. Infection control has been a 'bolt-on extra' (Figure 5.2).

'Do as you've always done and you'll get what you've always got' – to make a difference now, infection control must move from this 'bolt-on extra' position to the place it belongs at the heart of corporate governance, within the scope of a Trust's balanced score card (Figure 5.3).

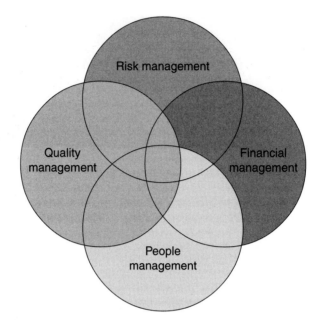

FIGURE 5.1 Corporate governance: the balanced score card.

Infection control

- Surveillance
- Decontamination
- Antibiotic control
- Bed management/
  patient admission/
  risk assessment
- Infection control/
  education and training
- Hand hygiene
- Infection control and
  personal development plan
- Directorate clinical
  governance improvement
- Estates and facilities
- Cleaning

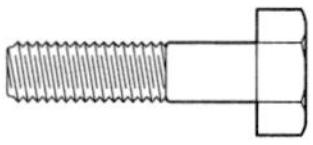

Corporate governance

FIGURE 5.2 Infection control as a 'bolt-on' extra to corporate governance.

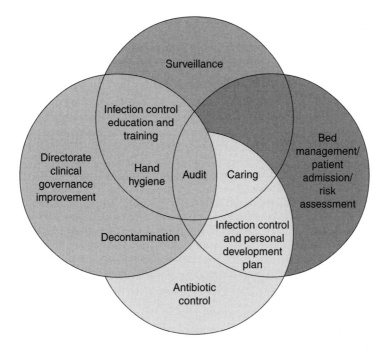

FIGURE 5.3 Infection control at the heart of corporate governance.

Clinical governance is a systematic approach to quality improvement

For a first-class service to be provided nationally, resources must be used efficiently, using standardized quality indicators that avoid unacceptable variations in services. To achieve this, improved standards and monitoring the approaches to quality improvement are a mandatory requirement.

Clinical governance may be viewed as a systematic approach to quality assurance and improvement within a clinical service, and there can be no better example of this than control of infection. We owe it to our patients to do our reasonable best to reduce all HCAI risks to which we expose them to an 'irreducible minimum', and yet, until recently, many Trusts had not even included infection incidents within their incident reporting system. Infection incidents have thus largely escaped organizational learning and have tended to occur again and again. This is of concern because, as the clinical governance process unfolds, improved quality care is now the expectation, in accordance with evidence-based clinical guidelines and evaluation of services through the use of tools such as clinical audit and clinical risk management, using outcome measures to further improve quality.

How do we know that what we are doing is right and how can we prove it?

Clinical governance is concerned with shifting the level of quality provided by the majority of healthcare organizations closer to the performance of the exemplar, which involves effective learning from leading-edge services. The public expects that clinical governance will be able to prevent the serious failures in standards of care which have occurred in the past. Healthcare organizations throughout the UK need to become learning organizations both of success and failure.

How do we know that what we are doing is wrong if we don't undertake the necessary surveillance, report incidents and learn from them?

Creating plans to address deficiencies in a service has become a vital part of the clinical governance process, and if it works well, there should be a *ripple effect* in the quality of care provided across the country. Clinical governance is above all about changing organizational culture in a systematic and demonstrable way, moving from a culture of 'blame' to one of learning so that quality infuses into all aspects of an organization's work.

Harnessing the knowledge and expertise of staff is one of the cornerstones of quality improvement

Closing the gap between the quality of the present service and the desired new level of quality will inevitably mean the need to address workforce issues: harnessing the knowledge and expertise of staff is one of the cornerstones of quality improvement through clinical governance.

Costs are multidimensional

Costs to the hospital sector associated with HCAI risks are enormous, and while it is normally the financial impact that is quoted, the true picture is much more multidimensional.

Figure 5.4 illustrates that HCAI may have both financial and non-financial consequences. Indeed, the public's perception of a Trust is likely to become profoundly important as Patient Choice develops. Complaints, litigation, poor staff morale and lost bed days due to HCAI could be devastating if

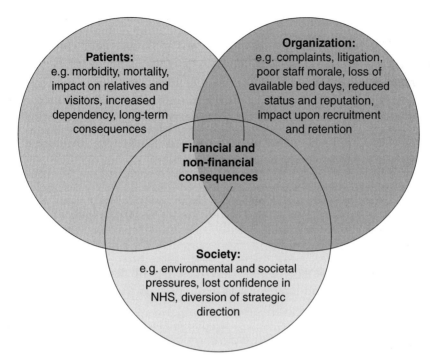

FIGURE 5.4 The risk management dimensions of healthcare-associated infection. Reproduced by kind permission of the *Journal of Hospital Infection*.

they result in a loss of public confidence. Indeed, we know that clean hospitals and the prevention of cross-infection *do* materially affect public confidence in the NHS, and the Government now advises that cleanliness is as important to the public as waiting times. According to the London Patient Choice project,[5] patients prioritize cleanliness over waiting times. A high quality of perceived care in relation to infection control is therefore vital and likely to influence the choice patients and their commissioners make about where to go for treatment.

HCAI presents a risk that must be managed

In risk management terms, HCAI presents a risk that must be managed. In recognizing this, the Department of Health has placed infection control in its first domain – quality – as a mandatory standard.[3]

Having placed infection control firmly within corporate governance and recognized the risk of infection for every patient, we now need to move on to comprehensively control this risk. Risk management is the process whereby risks are identified, assessed and controlled by asking the following questions:

- What is the right thing – what standards have been set?
- Are we doing the right thing – have we audited against these standards?
- How are we checking that we are doing it right – have we re-audited?

Answering these questions through the risk management agenda will enable Trusts to minimize or eradicate infection risks to patients, resulting in the quality of patient care being continuously raised.

The infection control delivery risks – What are the blocks?

A workshop held at the Autumn 2000 meeting of the Hospital Infection Society (HIS) reviewed infection control delivery in the UK at that time and identified the following operational risks:[6]

- lack of accountability of clinicians and managers
- ineffective surveillance with no ownership, resulting in infection problems not being identified
- problems identified and not being addressed through effective audit
- lack of communication and consultation by clinical teams
- lack of clear organizational links
- lack of organizational learning

Since this time, an additional risk has emerged, namely the conflict between high-quality infection control practice and Department of Health targets tending to increase bed occupancy and encourage movement of patients around the hospital.

One of the outcomes of the HIS Workshop was to identify the need to develop useful performance measures against which both performance and progress can be assessed.

Approaches to performance indicators in infection control

To support public ownership and awareness, an assessment framework is gradually being generated that places performance management against indicators at the heart of corporate governance on the national as well as the local stage. As time goes on, it is hoped that these indicators will become more meaningful and increasingly accurate.

The key to capturing clinical adoption and enthusiasm for performance indicators will be to ensure that those that are introduced are robust, informative and helpful in identifying and monitoring the actions that are needed.

There are at least three different types of indicators

1. *Structure indicators* that identify how closely national and/or local organizational rules are being followed and how an organization reflects these national or local rules. Structure indicators are usually evidenced by internal policies and guidelines that reflect compliance with statutory requirements. They have also been called 'compliance indicators'.
2. *Process indicators* indicate how people in the organization follow their own internal rules and guidelines, how they acquire knowledge about these rules and guidelines, and how they apply them. Examples could include how many people have access or attend internal (organizational) training courses or activities that show/teach how to implement these guidelines.

   Observational audit of specifically stated organizational requirements (e.g. hand hygiene activities following patient contact) may also be considered in this category.
3. *Outcome indicators* link a risk indicator to the progress of patients. These can indicate the performance of the organization against certain standards. Examples of this could be the rates of the HCAI among inpatients (e.g. urinary tract infection in catheterized patients or surgical site infections following clean surgery).

It is recognized that there is a natural tendency among clinicians to opt for this last type of indicator, as they most naturally reflect clinical experience and expectations.

Performance indicators and infection control

Although performance indicators are extensively used in industry, there is only now an awareness of the benefits that they can bring to the NHS.

All NHS Acute Trusts are now required to undertake direct laboratory reporting of specific quality-indicator organisms, including *Staphylococcus aureus* bacteraemia – both methicillin-sensitive *S. aureus* and methicillin-resistant *S. aureus* (MRSA) – *Clostridium difficile* diarrhoea and orthopaedic surgical site infections. Such indicators are reported nationally and Trusts are expected to move towards the performance of the best.

As indicated above, it is essential that infection control become part of corporate governance within the network of quality (controls assurance), people (clinical governance), risk management and financial management. As the clinical governance process develops, clinical effectiveness becomes the overarching tool to pull the different aspects of clinical governance together.

Clinical effectiveness is a process that may be considered as the right person doing:

- the right thing (evidence-based practice)
- in the right way (skills and competence)
- at the right time (providing treatment/services when patients need them)
- in the right place (location of treatment/services)
- with the right result (clinical effectiveness/maximizing health gain)

Surveillance and risk management must be at the centre of infection control strategy

Reflection of the above leads to a number of important conclusions. Firstly, surveillance and risk management must be at the centre of infection control practice and strategic development, with infection control teams, aligned operationally and organizationally to senior Trust managers, and with risk managers, in order to identify and prioritize developments.

Trusts must be able to demonstrate that their infection control services are effective and evidence-based. This can be achieved through targeted activities such as the surveillance of environmental standards and appropriate outcome measures. Trusts need to create a clear culture of personal responsibility and accountability among their staff in terms of their roles in protecting patients from the hazards of HCAI. This means that issues relating to infection control must be in all job descriptions and appraisal documents.

Clinicians must learn to become natural risk managers

In some aspects of professional practice, clinicians behave for the benefit of their patient as natural risk takers. This approach has no place in the prevention of HCAI, where clinicians must learn to become natural risk managers.

As an organization, the NHS has been poor at ensuring that demonstrable good practice in the service is systematically adopted widely. The lost opportunities to improve quality because of this weakness are enormous and known only too well to infection control teams. We are now well rehearsed in the statistics of HCAI and know that inpatients suffering these events result in an estimated 5000 deaths per annum, with an annual cost to the NHS of around £1 billion.[7]

A culture needs to be developed within Trusts in which lessons learnt from clinical audit programmes, from adverse event monitoring and 'near-miss reporting', and from patient feedback and complaints, as well as desired quality improvements and continuing health needs assessment, are routinely and explicitly translated into action.

NHS and the learning organization

Good practice, ideas and innovation need to be widely disseminated and seamlessly adopted. This requires an explicit recognition of the role of research and development, including mechanisms for reviewing evidence. This needs to be an open and transparent process, which seeks a partnership with other stakeholders, including the general public, involving them with the organization and delivery of services and the monitoring of performance.

Directorates now hold full management responsibility for all resources: financial, staff, equipment and facilities of the clinical specialty. They are held accountable to the Trust Board for the quality of clinical practice delivered, including control of infection. Learning lessons from the past is now an integral part of this process.

The Trust Board has the ultimate responsibility for ensuring that quality systems have been implemented and are maintained and developed, and must ensure that such systems are based on clear standards, as outlined in *Winning Ways*.[1] This document represents an autocratic instruction to Chief Executives to adopt national clinical guidelines with the objective of instilling an uncompromising commitment into managerial and clinical leadership. Such wholesale adoption of National Guidelines[8] is aimed at minimizing current inconsistencies in the UK. Where the evidence base is unproven, the opinion of the majority will be accepted.

Implementation of *Winning Ways*

Winning Ways was introduced in December 2003,[1] the key requirements being:

- Action Area One: active surveillance and investigation
- Action Area Two: reducing the infection risk from use of catheters, tubes, cannulae, instruments and other devices

- Action Area Three: reducing reservoirs of infection
- Action Area Four: high standards of hygiene in clinical practice
- Action Area Five: prudent use of antibiotics
- Action Area Six: management and organization
- Action Area Seven: research and development

Action Area One: active surveillance and investigation

Information drives action

In keeping with high-quality risk management, incident reporting and feedback of relevant and useful information to clinical teams is essential. It is time for clinical teams to have access to team-specific information on good practice through high-quality surveillance and be prompted to look critically at their own team practice of infections that occur. Such infections will include healthcare-associated *S. aureus* bacteraemia, *C. difficile* diarrhoea and surgical site wound infections.

A useful approach to dealing with such infections is the use of root-cause analysis by directorate management teams, who produce action plans to prevent recurrence. Complaints and deaths related to HCAI will also need investigating.

As part of the surveillance process, it is recommended that acute Trusts participate in the national Nosocomial Infection Surveillance Unit (NINSS) programme of surgical site wound infection. The categories of surgical procedures included in the surveillance are:

- hip hemiarthroplasty
- total hip
- total knee
- open reduction of long-bone fracture
- abdominal hysterectomy
- bile duct, liver or pancreatic surgery
- cholecystectomy, without exploration of bile duct (non-laparoscopic)
- coronary artery bypass graft (CABG)
- gastric surgery: incision, excision or anastomosis of stomach, partial or total gastrectomy, vagotomy, pyloromyotomy, pyloroplasty, and gastroenterostomy
- large-bowel surgery, including procedures that involve anastomosis of the small to the large bowel
- Limb amputation, including digits
- Small-bowel surgery, excluding anastomosis of the small to the large bowel

- Vascular surgery, excluding varicose veins repair, creation of arterial shunts, CABG or any procedure involving the pulmonary artery

Each clinical team will need equipping with the necessary tools to conduct the surveillance relevant to their practice, with epidemiological analysis of the results. This will enable factors associated with infection to be identified. Once identified, a team plan for controlling the risk can be developed. Performance management of this plan will need to be built into the Trust's top-level performance management arrangements. This approach exemplifies the balanced score card approach outlined above, with Trusts needing to invest in resources required to undertake this properly and, in doing so, expecting to make significant savings from reducing infection, while improving the quality of patient care.

Action Area Two: reducing the infection risk from use of catheters, tubes, cannulae, instruments and other devices

Trusts need to put in place systems to ensure that the following devices are only used in full accordance with National Guidelines:

- urinary catheters
- peripheral intravenous cannulae
- intravenous feeding lines
- central venous lines
- respiratory support devices

Adequate decontamination processes are implicit in the systems, which require developing.

Each directorate or clinical team will be required to provide evidence of implementation by regular audit, with action plans to correct non-compliances. Such audit will inform clinical governance improvement plans.

Action Area Three: reducing reservoirs of infection

The risks of HCAI are greatly increased by extensive movement of patients within the hospital, by very high bed occupancy and by an absence of suitable facilities to isolate infected patients.

Trusts need to arrange for bed managers to assess the impact of infection prior to each admission, with evidence that this has occurred. Appropriate admission, including the possible use of isolation facilities, will then be allocated.

Clinical teams need to ensure that visits by infected patients to other departments are preplanned and the risk is assessed and managed. Visiting also represents a profoundly important reservoir of infection, which requires controlling in a comprehensive way.

- Infection control staff need to be part of the teams overseeing plans for rebuilding and refurbishing work and setting contracts for services such as laundry and cleaning.
- NHS Trust Chief Executives need to ensure that the hospital environment is visibly clean, free from dust and soiling, and acceptable to patients, their visitors and staff.
- Cleaning and disinfecting programmes and protocols for environmental surfaces in patient care areas will be defined and carefully monitored to ensure that high standards of cleanliness are achieved.
- The segregation, handling, transport and disposal of waste needs to be properly managed so as to minimize the risks to the health and safety of staff, patients, the public and the environment, as set out in the relevant controls assurance standard.
- Infection control requirements will be designed-in at the planning stages of healthcare facilities, including new builds or renovation projects.
- Attention needs to be paid to the prevention of airborne infection by the use of ventilation in specialist areas and correct engineering and mechanical services.
- All healthcare settings need to aim to eradicate insect, bird and rodent pests such as rats, mice, ants, cockroaches, pigeons and flies.
- Contamination of the water supply in hospitals with bacteria such as *Legionella* needs to be avoided by appropriate building design and maintenance, cleaning water storage tanks, maintaining consistently high temperature in hot water supplies, keeping cold water systems cold, and minimizing water storage.
- All catering facilities in healthcare settings need to comply with current food safety legislation. This includes catering management, food handlers and premises from where food is sourced, stored, prepared or served.

Directorates need to undertake regular environmental audit, with action plans and progress against action plans. Demonstrable improvement in the quality of patient care should be evidenced over time through directorate governance improvement.

Action Area Four: high standards of hygiene in clinical practice

Healthcare workers are a major route by which patients become infected; microorganisms are transmitted by staff from one patient to another or from the environment to the patient:

- Each clinical team needs to demonstrate consistently high levels of compliance with handwashing and hand disinfection protocols.
- Clinical teams need to demonstrate consistently high standards of aseptic technique: for instance, by ensuring that all appropriate sterile items are available, that the setting is prepared and that manipulation of the affected site is minimized.
- Gloves, masks and protective clothing of an approved standard need to be used in every appropriate clinical care situation and properly disposed of after use. Used sharps will be disposed of in a sharps container at the place of use.
- Clinical teams need to rigorously adopt standard (universal) precautions to minimize the transmission of infection, including bloodborne viruses.
- Clinical teams need to ensure that if any additional infection control precautions are necessary, these are documented in patients' records.
- Induction programmes for all staff, including agency and locum staff, need to include local guidance on infection control and the use of aseptic technique.
- Infection control should be considered as part of the personal development plans for all healthcare staff.
- All appropriate healthcare staff need to be up to date with immunizations for hepatitis B, tuberculosis, influenza and chickenpox. Occupational health departments will ensure that healthcare workers are given the necessary health assessment and advice so that those known to be infected with bloodborne viruses do not carry out procedures that pose a risk of infection to patients.

Clinical teams will be expected to undertake regular hand hygiene audit, with action plans and progress against action plans. Demonstrable improvement in the quality of patient care should be evidenced over time through directorate and clinical team governance improvement.

Evidence of clinical team induction and ongoing education of infection control should be evidenced and included in directorate and clinical team action plans. This involves the inclusion of infection control in each individual's personal development plan within the Trust appraisal process.

Action Area Five: prudent use of antibiotics

Indiscriminate and inappropriate use of antibiotics to treat infection within a clinical service promotes the emergence of antibiotic-resistant organisms and the 'superbug' strains.

- Antibiotics will normally be used after a treatable infection has been recognized or there is a high degree of suspicion of infection.
- Choice of antibiotic will normally be governed by local information about trends in antibiotic resistance or a known sensitivity of the organism.
- Antibiotics will only be taken by patients over the prescribed period at the correct dose.
- Prescription of antibiotics for children will be carefully considered; they are often unnecessarily prescribed for common viral infections, and the child is subsequently more likely to develop a resistant infection.
- Support for prudent antibiotic prescribing in hospitals will be provided by the clinical pharmacists, medical microbiologists and infectious disease physicians on the staff.
- Antibiotics will be used for prevention of infection only where benefit has been proven.
- Narrow-spectrum antibiotics will be preferred to the broad-spectrum groups.

Directorates and clinical teams will regularly audit their use of antibiotics against Trust Standards. Demonstrable improvement in the quality of patient care should be evidenced over time through directorate governance improvement.

Action Area Six: management and organization

Tackling HCAI cannot be left to clinical staff alone; senior management commitment, local infrastructure and systems are also vital.

- Chief Executives of NHS Trusts and Primary Care Trusts will designate the prevention and control of HCAI as a core part of their organization's clinical governance and patient safety programmes.
- Chief Executives of NHS organizations will be aware of factors within organizations that promote low levels of HCAI and ensure that the appropriate action is taken.
- Chief Executives of NHS organizations will be aware of their legal duties to identify, assess and control risks of infection in the workplace.

- A Director of Infection Prevention and Control will be designated within each organization providing NHS services, and will:
  - oversee local control of infection policies and their implementation
  - be responsible for the infection control team within the healthcare organization
  - report directly to the Chief Executive and the Board and not through any other officer
  - have the authority to challenge inappropriate clinical hygiene practice as well as antibiotic-prescribing decisions
  - assess the impact of all existing and new policies and plans on infection and make recommendations for change
  - be an integral member of the organization's clinical governance and patient safety teams and structures
  - produce an annual report on the state of HCAI in the organization(s) for which he/she is responsible and release it publicly
- The Department of Health will publish further guidance on the roles and responsibilities of infection control teams.
- The Department of Health will work with the Royal Colleges and professional regulatory bodies to ensure that strong emphasis is given to infection control in the undergraduate and postgraduate curricula of nursing, medical, dental and other healthcare students and trainees.
- The Department of Health will ensure that its expertise and specialist agencies are made available to facilitate change and improvement in local NHS facilities; the Clinical Governance Support Team, the Modernisation Agency, the National Patient Safety Agency, the new Inspector of Microbiology and the Health Protection Agency all have key roles in this respect.
- The Department of Health (with NHS Direct, the National Patient Safety Agency and the Patient Advice and Liaison Services) will ensure that up-to-date information is provided to the public/patients on infection control and how HCAI can be prevented.
- Strategic Health Authorities will be accountable for ensuring that NHS performance management arrangements are aligned to achieve the objectives of this report. As part of their local audit programmes, NHS Trusts and Primary Care Trusts will include assessment of adherence to standard (universal) precautions to reduce the transmission of HCAI.
- The Healthcare Commission will be asked to give priority to assessing NHS performance in reducing HCAI.

Action Area Seven: research and development

Evidence and experience

The control of HCAI and of the commonest of the multiresistant bacteria, MRSA, is a major concern of many health services in the world.

The level of HCAI among patients who are hospitalized in the USA, Australasia and most European countries is between 4% and 10% (Table 5.1). Data on levels of MRSA bloodstream infections as a proportion of all *S. aureus* bloodstream infections show that the UK is among those with the highest levels in Europe (Table 5.2).

Most countries are adopting similar strategies to control HCAI, based upon:

- developing high-quality surveillance systems
- setting clear standards for infection control
- majoring on clean hospital environments and good hygiene practice
- strict antibiotic-prescribing policies
- isolating infected patients in side-rooms or cubicles
- making HCAI a key feature of quality and patient safety programmes

Some countries have been particularly successful in controlling MRSA. The experience of the Netherlands is notable. The Dutch strategy has been based on a policy of 'search and destroy'. This involves screening patients for MRSA and isolating those found to be positive (colonized or infected). The Dutch have been able to set aside sufficient numbers of single rooms in

TABLE 5.1 Estimated prevalence of healthcare-associated infection

USA	5–10%	Denmark	8%
Australia	6%	France	6–10%
Norway	7%	Netherlands	7%
England	9%	Spain	8%

Source: Thames Valley University, Richard Wells Research Centre and other expert sources.

TABLE 5.2 Proportion of *Staphylococcus aureus* blood isolates resistant to methicillin (i.e. MRSA)

Denmark	1%	France	33%
Netherlands	1%	Portugal	38%
Austria	11%	Italy	38%
Germany	19%	Greece	44%
Spain	23%	UK	44%

Source: European Antimicrobial Resistance Surveillance System data for 2002.

modern hospitals and maintain a high healthcare worker-to-patient ratio. As a result, this approach has been remarkably successful. The proportion of *S. aureus* bloodstream isolates resistant to methicillin among hospital patients in the Netherlands is 1%.

Implementation and performance management: clarity of roles and accountabilities

The Health and Safety at Work Act 1974 places duties on employers to ensure, as far as is reasonably practicable, that they do not expose their employers to risks of health and safety while they are at work. This duty of employers also extends to persons not in their employment, including patients and members of the public. Now that the Department of Health has identified infection control in the first domain of their core standards, it is incumbent on Trusts to urgently relook at their infection control arrangements, ultimate responsibility for effective arrangements lying with the Chief Executive, who is accountable to the Department of Health.

Achieving the approach

At the heart of achieving the above approach is the need to gain clinical leadership and ownership of the process, while ensuring that these individuals have the tools to do the job, including accurate, useful and timely surveillance upon which appropriate initiatives can be based and monitored.

Embedding infection control in the heart of corporate governance should allow appropriate strategic priorities to be resourced. For example, the cost-effectiveness of surveillance systems and the effective transfer of data into information for action should become fully realized.

As the system unfolds, the Healthcare Commission will be assessing the performance of Trusts against the implementation of *Winning Ways* and in accordance with *Standards for Better Health*.

Infection control practitioners should welcome this approach and over the next few years, HCAI should be truly reduced to that irreducible minimum.

References

1. *Winning Ways*: working together to reduce healthcare associated infection in England (December 2003): http://www.dh.gov.uk/assetRoot/04/06/46/89/04064689.pdf.

2. Towards cleaner hospitals and lower rates of infection (July 2004): http://www.dh.gov.uk/assetRoot/04/08/58/61/04085861.pdf.
3. Standards for Better Health (July 2004): http://www.dh.gov.uk/assetRoot/04/08/66/66/04086666.pdf.
4. The Matron's Charter: an action plan for cleaner hospitals (October 2004): http://www.dh.gov.uk/assetRoot/04/09/15/07/04091507.pdf.
5. Rand Europe, Kings Fund and City University 2003/4: www.londonchoice.nhs.uk/othertopics-patientdecision.php.
6. Masterton R, Teare L, Richards J. Hospital Infection Society/Association of Medical Microbiologists 'Towards a Consensus II' Workshop I: Hospital-acquired infection and risk management. *J Hosp Infect* 2002; **51**: 17–20.
7. Plowman R, Graves N, Griffin M *et al. The Socio-economic Burden of Hospital Acquired Infection.* London: Public Health Laboratory Service/London School of Hygiene and Tropical Medicine, 1999.
8. The EPIC Project: Developing National Evidence Based Guidelines for Preventing Healthcare Associated Infection. *J Hosp Infect* 2001: **47**(Suppl).

6

Accurate clinical information: From myth to reality?

Nicola Roderick

With the introduction of the concept of clinical governance in the Government White Paper *The New NHS: Modern, Dependable*[1] in 1997 came the recognition that the NHS would have to find ways to better utilize 'clinical information'.

In secondary care Trusts at that time, such information was not always available, was not always accurate, and was rarely owned by the clinicians. There were many problems surrounding information and data that needed to be resolved in order to fully support the clinical governance process, and to shift the focus of patient information from being a management and financial tool towards an electronic patient record (EPR). It was widely recognized that changes were needed in the very culture of the NHS, and that investment was urgently needed.

A number of high-profile enquiries had shown that long-ingrained information problems have undermined the quality of care.[2] The Kennedy Report on paediatric cardiac surgery was critical of information systems in use to monitor clinical performance.[3]

While the Kennedy Report encouraged extending the use of the Health Episode Statistics (HES) data collected from trusts in England, there are doubts as to

> 'whether the data are fit for all the purposes to which they are now being put. In particular, a much higher standard of accuracy is needed if decisions are to be based on information from relatively small local data sets that can easily be distorted by a few significant errors.'[3]

Although the ultimate goal of a fully integrated EPR will take many years for all Trusts to achieve; the governmental strategies of the last few years are starting to evaluate the scale of the problem. The Strategy for NHS Information Quality Assurance[4] points out that 'whilst there are many individual examples of excellence, it is clear that in general the quality of much of the data held within NHS systems remains inadequate.'

What does clinical governance need?

Clinical governance needs good-quality data and information. This is essential in two realms:

- In face-to-face contacts with patients, it is necessary to ensure that the clinical decisions are properly informed, with all possible data being available to the clinician. The National Patient Safety Agency (NPSA), established in 2001 to collect information on adverse health events, has made it clear that poor information quality can contribute to such events.[5] Indeed, the Welsh Information Strategy, *Informing Healthcare*, states that 'If we can integrate patient information then we can integrate patient care'.[2]
- It is essential to ensure that aggregate information can be used for clinical audit, making decisions on best clinical practice, and enabling medical and clinical directors to assess the performance of clinicians. The new arrangements for the appraisals of consultants will necessitate the production of evidence of good medical practice. Peer comparison and benchmarking will inevitably form part of that, and this will not be possible without good-quality data and information.

Data routinely collected from Trusts across England and Wales have already been used to compare performance through clinical indicators and NHS performance reporting.

What information is currently available?

Within an average acute hospital Trust, there is no shortage of patient-based data. The primary source of this will be the patient administration system (PAS). This relatively complex dataset will manage a patient through from GP referral to treatment, including waiting lists and outpatient appointments. Medical records staff, ward clerks and clinical coders will enter data. This data set will be designed around national standards and definitions. The APC (admitted patient care) dataset will be at its core, and data for inpatients and day cases should therefore be comparable with that for Trusts, data quality permitting. The more clinically useful aspect of the dataset is the ICD-10 and OPCS-4 codes added by the clinical coding staff to inpatient episodes and day-case records. These are derived from patients' medical records based upon the documented diagnoses and procedures carried out.

Acute Trusts actually have a wealth of other information sources, such as theatre systems, pathology systems, X-ray and probably a host of 'local' clinical systems to support particular specialties or conditions. These systems may not all be based on national standards and data definitions, and while the quality of resulting data may be good within its own definitions, it is unlikely to be comparable with other data.

Other data that prove useful for clinical governance will be found in incident, complaints and claim management systems. Certainly, the collection of data about clinical incidents centrally as part of the National Reporting and Learning System (NRLS) at the NPSA will bring comparability to such data by providing common definitions and structures to the data. From a clinical governance point of view, analysis of the issues that arise from incidents and their underlying causes may be useful to prevent recurrence. Through the NRLS, lessons learned in one Trust can theoretically be passed on to all others.

Where is the problem?

Most Trusts have many different information systems that have been developed in a piecemeal fashion as needs have arisen over many years. The PAS and systems for areas such as theatres, radiology, pathology and pharmacy have been purchased separately from different suppliers. Many smaller systems were often bought or created to support the needs of individual specialities/services. Such systems do not always contain standard patient identifiers or national data definitions, and are used in isolation from each other. The compatibility problems that arise from this situation are compounded by Trust mergers and reconfigurations, which increase the numbers of systems in use within one organization.

This fragmentation leads to duplication of input and creates a huge administrative problem – trying to keep all these systems synchronized. If a change of address or name is received, or even a notification of death, it needs to be reflected in all such systems. It is likely that staff do not know about the other systems that need to be updated.

While most Trusts are not in a position to replace all their legacy systems, there has been a growing recognition over the years of the need to ensure that all new patient-based systems (and old ones where possible) should be linked to a common patient master index (PMI) – usually that contained within the PAS. Any changes to details for a patient need to be made in the pivotal system and cascaded through to the other systems. This guarantees the consistency and quality of demographics in all such systems, and should help to avoid those painful scenarios where a patient does not receive an appointment letter because it has been sent to the wrong address, or correspondence is sent to deceased patients. But there are other benefits.

This PMI can be used as the core of a virtual EPR, linking many data sources and making them available to a much wider audience through one seamless interface. The 'Technical Proof of Concept' project in Wales[5] has explored possible approaches to a single record, including the use of data repositories and the problems surrounding the use of perhaps unstructured data from legacy systems.

But while this is undoubtedly technically possible, even a virtual EPR is no use without a PC on every consultant's desk, or available in the areas where the clinical staff work. Investment is needed in IT throughout each Trust, and all staff involved in clinical care have to be given a basic education in the use of IT – whether or not they want it. The world is changing.

How do we measure data quality?

Good-quality data must be complete, accurate and timely. It is relatively straightforward to perform checks to make sure that fields are populated with valid codes and that those codes are compatible with other codes recorded. What is more difficult to ascertain is whether or not the correct information has been recorded.

> 'Considerable attention has also been focussed upon readily measurable aspects of data quality, namely the validity and completeness of data items, whilst harder to measure but perhaps more important aspects in the context of overall information quality, such as accuracy, have been neglected.'

> *A Strategy for NHS Information Quality Assurance*[4]

The following issues will probably have become familiar to most Trusts over the years, and some of these issues will be difficult to eliminate completely:

- duplicate patient records
- failure to transfer patients between consultants
- incorrect usage of codes
- failure to identify that a patient has died
- overlooked episodes
- incorrect admission, transfer or discharge dates
- failure to relate elective admissions to the WL entries they resulted from

The resolution of these problems will rely on a combination of robust procedures and staff education (including that of clinical staff) about their role and responsibilities in the data collection process. While some of the above quality issues cannot be deduced from the data, others, such as failure to transfer, can emerge while benchmarking. A coronary artery bypass graft performed by a cardiologist usually raises eyebrows! However, it can be difficult to see the wood for the trees when shared care is not adequately recorded in the datasets.

The practical difficulties of data quality

Controlling the quality of information is a task that should not be underestimated. While everyone pays lip service to the importance of good-quality information, there is a great reluctance to resource information collection functions adequately and to act upon identified problems and errors. Education, communication and ownership at all levels of the organization are essential to facilitate cultural change.

Both the Audit Commission[3] and the Commission for Health Improvement (CHI) have commented on the poor quality of data found in their reviews at some Trusts. While there has always been a broad agreement on the importance of collecting accurate data, there also seems to be a common perception within many Trusts that it is somebody else's problem. In reality, such problems can be due to:

- failure of Trust management to take such issues seriously
- grade of staff inputting data
- staff with other priorities
- failure to train staff adequately
- inadequate system front-end validation
- failure to make information available for inputting

The *Strategy for NHS Information Quality Assurance* suggests that we should consider whether the sort of failings mentioned above are the errors of individuals or 'part of a more pervasive organisational failing'.[4]

At corporate level, there is often a failure to understand how difficult it is to collect even the relatively simple data contained in the standard minimum datasets accurately. Hospitals are very complex environments, and patients can have many different entry and exit points to the system. How does a Trust ensure that *every* patient who comes through the door has their demographic and GP details checked and any amendments entered onto the central system? How do you track all ward and consultant changes? Given the complexity of healthcare, it is perhaps surprising that the data is as accurate as it is! All of these complexities have to be taken into account when setting up the processes for collection of the data and ensuring that the right data is recorded first time.

However, the quality of data is dependent upon the staff responsible for input. They are not always sufficiently educated in the importance and uses of the data, leading to the tendency to use 'bucket' codes or even to misuse fields. The system is a 'black box' into which data is input, and they do not see what is extracted from it. Errors can go on for years and be discovered quite by accident.

Even the apparently simple task of recording events against the correct patient record can be difficult. Patients seldom arrive brandishing their NHS number, and the elderly, not very lucid or unconscious may be unable to give their names. Patients may legally have one name but use another. Add a change of address since last admission, or an error in birth date, and they look like a completely different person. This can potentially lead to multiple records – both paper and electronic. Although it may not be possible to avoid all of these errors at the point of contact, Trusts must have procedures for identifying and merging such records.

Only trained staff should be inputting data. They should be informed of the importance of data quality, and the consequences of getting it wrong. They need to know what procedures are in place when information is difficult to obtain. Of course, the need for data may appear to compete with the needs of patients and look relatively unimportant. Sometimes, the information necessary for input to the system is not available at input time, or ward clerks are not informed when a patient changes ward or consultant. There is also a continual expectation at management level that additional data can be recorded without any increase in staffing level.

Whatever systems are used for collecting data, they must have appropriate front-end validation controls to ensure that conflicting data or nonsense data cannot be entered. For example, a patient who has died cannot have a discharge destination of home. Input screens should be clear, unambiguous and easy to read. Bucket codes and default values should be eliminated where possible. Systems should produce regular exception reports on data that are subjective or anomalous, for review. There should be an audit trail for every data item. Errors should be traced back for correction and education – users can then learn from their mistakes.

The Audit Commission's *Data Remember* document[3] states that the improvement of data quality needs to become a higher priority. It also points out the 'Catch 22' of data quality:

> 'The biggest obstacle to data quality over all is that information systems are not all actively used. A system that is well used is likely to improve.'

Making timely data available to clinical staff is an excellent form of audit. Clinicians know whether or not they have cared for a certain patient, or undertaken a certain procedure. However, it is difficult to engage clinicians when using a system widely known to have inaccurate data. If the errors and anomalies that they point out are not dealt with, their interest and enthusiasm will rapidly wane.

Dead or alive

Currently collected data are of limited use when trying to measure the quality of care that patients receive while in hospital. The standard minimum dataset only identifies whether or not a patient has died in hospital, and to where they have been discharged (i.e. home, nursing home or another NHS acute hospital). A day-surgery patient dying at home of a pulmonary embolism three days postoperatively would not be recorded on the hospital information system. It is difficult for clinicians to know that such patients have died at all, let alone that their death is perhaps related to their treatment.

The identification of patient deaths outside a Trust is a constant headache. While there is media outrage when the relatives of a deceased patient receive an appointment letter, it is seldom reported that the hospital cannot know this unless they are told! The administrative death registers used in England and Wales can take weeks or months to be updated, as they are based on information reported by GP practices. These then have to be matched with a Trust's PMI – an exercise that cannot be carried out reliably by an algorithm without informed human intervention. While the increasing population of NHS numbers should help this process, being absolutely sure that the John Smith that died last week is the John Smith you currently have recorded on database (especially if he has outstanding appointments) is essential from a clinical point of view, and extremely sensitive from the patient's point of view.

Clinicians would like to know more than if their patients survive! It would be useful to know if their patients' quality of life has improved, and whether or not the treatment administered was effective. They should be able to audit the outcomes of various forms of treatments to decide whether or not they are effective and worthwhile. This can be achieved by sending out audit questionnaires to patients who have been discharged (after checking for deceased patients). However, the processing and analysis of such data is relatively labour-intensive since it is project-based and not routinely collected.

The attribution of deaths is viewed very simplistically in the datasets. As each record is a consultant episode, the last consultant to have an episode in the patient spell of care is the one generally accepted to be 'responsible' for the death. However, this could be a surgeon or intensivist taking over a failing patient from another clinician. The dataset could also mask procedures involving multiple surgeons – for example, a patient dying of stroke after carotid endarterectomy simultaneous with coronary bypass surgery would almost certainly be attributed to the cardiac surgeon. In fact, contributory factors to a surgical patient's death could be the anaesthetist, physiotherapist, theatre staff or the postoperative nursing team, but there are practically no data collected in these areas. The outcome for the patient is only as good as the efforts of the team. It is extremely simplistic to label one consultant for things he/she may have no control over. Crude mortality rates also mask the fact that some clinicians treat patients with several comorbidities whose likelihood of mortality or poor outcome is high.

Clinical coding

Clinical coding refers to the part of the admitted patient care dataset that records patients' diagnoses and procedures. It is added to inpatient and day-case patient records by trained clinical coding staff interpreting information written in the patient's notes by the clinicians, and translating it into the ICD-10 and OPCS-4 coding systems.

The standard classifications

'Clinical coding' is perhaps a misleading term. The mandatory coding systems of OPCS-4 (Classification of Surgical Operations and Procedures) and ICD-10 (International Statistical Classification of Diseases and Related Health Problems) in current usage in minimum datasets are statistical rather than clinical. However, such classifications followed properly do allow the comparison of data collected in various hospitals, and do provide some information about the care of a patient in a hospital. While they may not suit every area, they are not without use. They can be used to analyse clinical care, even though this analysis may be limited.

OPCS-4 is a four-digit alphanumeric classification. Each code has an alpha prefix, which identifies either the whole or part of a body system – for example, 'C' is *Eye*, 'G' *is Upper Digestive Tract* and 'W' is *Other Bones and Joints*. The first three digits give a general description of the type of procedure (e.g. 'W06' is *Total excision of bone*). The final digit identifies the procedure more specifically (e.g. 'W06.5' is *Total excision of bone of foot nec.*). Most three-digit classifications include 'Other specified' and 'Unspecified' subcategorizations.[7] There are around 6000 codes altogether.

ICD-10 is mainly a four-digit alphanumeric classification. Each describes either a particular body systems diseases/disorders *Diseases of respiratory system*) or a type of disease/disorder ..g. ~ ιs *Neoplasms* and 'F' is *Mental and behavioural disorders*). The first three digits give a general description of the type of disease/disorder (e.g. 'J44' is *Other chronic obstructive pulmonary disease*). The fourth digit then further identifies the disease (e.g. 'J440' is *Chronic obstructive pulmonary disease with acute lower respiratory infection*). Again there are usually 'Other specified' and 'Unspecified' subcategories available.[7]

Many clinicians do not like to use the above classifications, finding them restrictive and unfamiliar. The development of Clinical Terms (Read codes) allows the capture of diagnostic and procedural information from a clinical perspective, which can then be translated back into ICD-10 and OPCS-4. Clinical Terms not only hold codes for diseases and operations, but also encompass clinical findings and presenting symptoms. Clinical Terms Version 3 is due to be introduced as the standard for operational clinical systems in the UK and is supported by *Information for Health*.[8]

There are plans to ensure international comparability in the future. SNOMED Clinical Terms is a joint development by the NHS and the College of American Pathologists (CAP), and will combine SNOMED RT (CAP's Systematized Nomenclature of Medicine – Reference Terminology) and Clinical Terms Version 3. This is intended to become an essential component of EPR.

ICD-10 and OPCS-4 are rapidly approaching 15 years of age. Since they were published, practice has moved on, with new conditions being diagnosed and new procedures (e.g. laser surgery) being carried out. Amendments to ICD-10 have been issues over the last few years, but there are very few new codes. However, coders are restricted to the classifications, and therefore have to make the best match for a particular diagnosis/condition. It is interesting to note that there is no specific ICD-10 code for the extremely newsworthy methicillin-resistant *Staphylococcus aureus* (MRSA). As Clinical Terms maps back to these classifications, accuracy in analysis will continue to be affected.

Coding quality

The use of the OPCS-4 and ICD-10 coding classifications is mandatory in the admitted patient care minimum datasets of Trusts' PAS. However, the process of correctly collecting and recording such information is fraught with difficulty.

The staff responsible for recording events and diagnoses in the patient notes are usually busy junior doctors, rather than their more experienced consultant colleagues. Those writing in the patient notes do not always understand the significance of such information for other purposes. Events/diagnoses can go unrecorded, or if present are often recorded illegibly. Sometimes, conflicting diagnoses are recorded without any further explanation. Bad filing can make it extremely difficult for coders to find enough information – in the worst-case scenarios, they sometimes have to code from scraps of paper. While coders have rigorous rules to follow about how they should code from the notes, clinical statements are not presented in a way that makes these rules easy to follow. Use of abbreviations can also cause confusion – meaning different things to different people. Notes may not be available because they have been sent to the coroner or are temporarily missing.

Not all coders find it easy to check or query comments in the notes with clinicians. There is usually little time to code each set of notes and no time to revisit the coding. Coding is often rushed to meet local and/or regional deadlines. Additional workload, such as the coding of outpatients/waiting lists, only adds to the pressures. This will inevitably affect the quality of the coding produced. In addition, coders are often based in obscure parts of the hospital, giving them little profile. Some clinical staff remain unaware of what the coders do or who they are.

In the past, the importance of having trained coders was not always understood. To ensure comparability between coded information everywhere, all coders need to be fully trained in the usage of ICD-10 and OPCS-4 and to keep up to date with central guidance and coding rules. They must always comply with the coding rules, and local deviations from recommended practice must be avoided. Pick lists should be outlawed, and the use of unspecified codes monitored carefully. Coders must ensure that they do code all relevant comorbidities to ensure that the complexity of patients is accurately reflected. However, it is important also to ensure that they do not 'overcode' a record by including conditions relating to an earlier episode that have no bearing on the management of the patient in the current episode. They should avoid coding signs and symptoms rather than diagnoses.

There is a need for consistency in coding between coders within a Trust and between Trusts to ensure comparability of data. Quality indicators must be monitored within each Trust, and used as indicators of relative coding quality between Trusts. Typical, if somewhat crude, indicators of coding quality are:

- average number of codes per episode
- the frequency of 'ungroupable' DRG (Diagnosis Related Group) or HRG (Healthcare Resource Group) codes
- the incidence of unspecified/non-specified codes, i.e. not coding to the required level of specificity
- the use of signs and symptoms codes as primary diagnoses

However, while such coding may appear to be technically corr
independent audit can be the ultimate guarantor of coding
comparability. Trusts in England and Wales are starting to make ....iprocal
arrangements to audit coding in the absence of a central audit function.

There has also been debate as to whether or not clinical staff themselves
should be coding. While it is arguable that they would know exactly what
happened to the patients, they would also have to submit to coding discipline
to ensure consistency within and between Trusts. There is no room for 'doing
your own thing', and evidence to date suggests that conformity does not rest
easy with clinicians.

The coding profession

According to the Audit Commission Report *Data Remember*,[3] clinical coding
is largely a graduate profession in the USA and Australia. This is not the case
in the UK, where coders' remuneration is often on a par with secretaries or
lower. The introduction over the last five years or so of a recognized coding
qualification is helping to advance the profession.

It takes around six months of constantly having their work checked by an
experienced member of staff and a two-week training course to bring a new
coder up to the minimum standard required, so the retention of staff is
essential. Low rates of pay, coupled with the fact that not all Trusts give any
financial recognition when coders do achieve the national qualification, not
only act as a disincentive to work for the qualification, but in the longer term
will lead the more promising staff to look to develop their potential elsewhere!

Part of the necessary information culture change in the NHS does involve
building relationships between clinicians and the coding profession, and
providing opportunities for discussions about complex cases. The feedback of
coded information to clinicians should also raise awareness of coding
problems.

Inadequacies of the datasets

The APC minimum dataset is used across England and Wales for collecting
data for the HES and PEDW National Databases respectively for inpatient and
day-case activity. But the data items contained within have not changed since
the Korner review in the 1970s and fail to reflect current clinical working
practices.[3]

Most Trusts struggle today to fit their data into the restrictive minimum
datasets, and to extract useful information from them. Team working is not

reflected in consultant episodes, and difficulties arise when trying to record shared care. Sometimes, a medical team will have the ongoing care of a patient despite the fact that the patient is taken away to theatres to have a procedure. It then appears that a non-surgical team are engaging in surgery.

The evolution of anaesthetists into intensivists also causes problems. They can be understandably aggrieved when reports based on their Korner code show their activity as 'Anaethetics'. Secondly, because they are not always perceived as being the patient's consultant, they can appear to have little activity in the datasets. These issues are harder to resolve, as there are gradations in the amount of care they share with consultants who admitted some of these patients. Can there be agreement with their non-intensivist colleagues as to who is primarily responsible? There is an augmented dataset for recording this activity, however, it has not been implemented in Wales and is not always yet used in England.

From data to information?

> ' "Forty two!" yelled Loonquawl. Is that all you've got to show for seven and a half million years' work?"
>
> "I checked it very thoroughly," said the computer, "and that quite definitely is the answer. I think the problem, to be quite honest with you, is that you've never actually known what the question is."
>
> "But it was the Great Question! The Ultimate Question of Life, the Universe and Everything", howled Loonquawl.
>
> "Yes," said Deep Thought with the air of one who suffers fools gladly, "but what actually *is* it?" '
>
> *The Hitch Hiker's Guide to the Galaxy*[9]

It is important to understand that data and information are not the same thing. While poor-quality data will inevitably lead to poor-quality information, we cannot assume that good-quality data will necessarily lead to good-quality information!

There are five issues here:

- data quality
- common understanding – interpretation of data
- context/provenance
- asking the right questions!
- limitations of the dataset

It is not sufficient to have good data collection processes in place. Data are the raw material from which information is created, and there is much information produced that does not answer any questions or help the organization to progress. Many of the failures to turn data into information stem from communication problems embedded within the very culture of the organization.

Data are stored with very precise definitions of the various data items; however, these are not always understood to mean the same things by management, clinicians, information analysts and the data input staff. All parties have responsibility:

- The data input staff must be educated about what the data are used for.
- Those who input and extract the data must have a common understanding of how data are recorded.
- Analysts must be explicit when passing on information to clinicians and managers about the criteria used for extracting the data and any factors that influence the result.
- Clinicians and management must define their queries clearly and keep both the analysts and the data input staff informed about changes in working practice and new developments.

It is important to ask the right questions in order to get the information required. Sometimes, it appears that clinicians and managers expect to be given the right information when they do not actually know the question. There is often a 'Chinese whispers' approach to information requests. A senior manager or clinician asks their assistant to ask their secretary to ring the Information Department and ask for some information, without also passing along the understanding about why the information is needed or what it is expected to prove. The data that are produced do not answer the question, or prove the point, or do not fit the purpose. Either the producers of the information are blamed, or the data are (once again) ridiculed.

There is not only a need to ask the right questions, however. One of the major problems with interpreting information is putting it into context. It is important to know that half the beds on a ward were closed for a period of time when calculating occupancy levels. However, there are rarely formal mechanisms in place within the organization to ensure that the appropriate people are made aware of such events.

The widespread use of intranet technology allows the provision of user-friendly online tools and reports that can be used to view and analyse data – self-service solutions. While this will be a useful leverage for opening out the data and encouraging ownership, it must be clear to the end-users what it is that they have asked for so that they really understand how to interpret the results!!

The development of a common language and common understanding will be of the utmost importance when defining the EPR. As the ideal is to capture data at point of contact, this means that all clinicians, nursing staff and PAMs (Professions Allied to Medicine) must have an equivalent understanding of how their data are recorded, and exactly what they mean. The introduction of informatics qualifications and training should allow the permeation of such skills through the organization.

Contextual issues will become very important. Results-reporting systems are sometimes reluctant to allow their data to be broken down into fields, because the textual information that accompanies a test result is considered to be as important as whether or not it was positive or negative.

Benchmarking

Every clinician is aware that they should be comparing their activity with other clinical teams and other Trusts. However, the datasets can limit the usefulness of this.

HRGs should help to compare like resource groups, but sometimes they are not specific enough to be helpful. It is perhaps difficult to determine at what level it is useful to analyse.

Specialty comparisons with other Trusts can at first glance give cause for concern. If a specialty length of stay or mortality rate is significantly higher than that of the peer group, the data may require checking down to individual consultant level. In any one year, an individual surgeon will undertake statistically quite small numbers of a particular operation and it requires looking at three or preferably five years' worth of data in order to be able to draw any meaningful conclusions.

The more worrying converse scenario is that an overall acceptable or even good performance at specialty or HRG level may mask areas of concern. One consultant's exemplary results may counterbalance another's rather poor results. This, linked to some of the contextual issues, can make it difficult to draw conclusions. Even more frustrating, a worrying mortality statistic can be checked in detail and audited against patients' notes, yet still yield no clear conclusions. The surgery may have been exemplary yet the patient died from poor attention to fluid balance by nurses and shift-working junior doctors.

It is also important to note that contextual information can also affect the interpretation of data. For instance, acute Trusts able to decant certain groups of patients (e.g. fractured neck of femur) to community hospitals will have different length-of-stay profiles for such conditions compared with integrated Trusts who manage such patients through to discharge home. They may also show a reduced mortality rate.

Are we doing enough – Will it succeed?

The strategies in place across England and Wales are mapping out the path towards a robust EPR. Issues identified include poor data quality, previous low priority of such issues and lack of system integration.

Some of the issues, such as the relevance of the data collected, will have to be nationally determined. Others, such as data accuracy, will have to be dealt with by the individual Trusts using sound processes and data collection mechanisms, robust systems, and staff training.

What is not so clear is how Trusts get to from where they are to where they want to be. They have struggled to maintain data quality in limited, non-contextual datasets. How will they be able to guarantee '100% accuracy 100% of the time' – the desirable situation stated in the *Strategy for Information Quality Assurance*[5]? According to the Audit Commission documents,[3] the Trusts with the best record in data quality are those where this has become a corporate objective.

The scale of these problems must not be underestimated. While the goals have been identified and the strategies are setting out some of the frameworks within which we need to work to achieve these goals, the actual changes required by organizations in terms of both cultural and technical change is immense. There are issues embedded very deep in the culture of every Trust, such as the ownership of the data. Politically inspired health targets are usually relatively easy to measure – waiting times, the four-hour A&E wait – and thus Trusts invest time and energy measuring these 'outcomes' rather than investing in looking at more difficult quality-of-care measures. Investment is necessary not only in the IT infrastructure, but also in the staff to input the data and check its quality.

The old administrative systems were always seen as competing for resources with patient care. All Trusts now have to take the view that investment in the information infrastructure is an investment in patient care, and that information technology can help to deliver a better service for the patient.

References

1. *The New NHS: Modern, Dependable*. London: Department of Health, December 1997.
2. *Informing Healthcare. Transforming Healthcare Using Information and IT*. Cardiff: Welsh Assembly Government, July 2003.
3. *Data Remember. Improving the Quality of Patient-Based Information in the NHS*. London: Audit Commission, March 2002.

4. *Consultation Draft. A Strategy for NHS Information Quality Assurance*. London: Information Policy Unit, Department of Health, 22 March 2004.
5. *Single Integrated Electronic Health Record Technical Proof of Concept*. Informing Healthcare, January 2005.
6. *Tabular List of the Classification of Surgical Operations and Procedures, Fourth Revision*. London: Office of Population Censuses and Surveys, 1990.
7. *International Statistical Classification of Diseases and Related Health Problems, Tenth Revision*. Geneva: World Health Organization 1990.
8. *Information for Health. An Information Strategy for the Modern NHS 1998–2005*. London: NHS Executive.
9. Adams D. *The Hitch Hiker's Guide to the Galaxy*. London: Pan, 1979.

Further reading

Clinical Coding Manual. London: NHS Executive, September 2000.
Working Together with Health Information. A Partnership Strategy for Education, Training and Development. London: NHS Executive, December 1999.
Building the Information Core – Implementing the NHS Plan. London: Department of Health, 2001.

7 The nursing and midwifery contribution to clinical governance

Anna Maslin, John Miller and Edward Griffiths

In developing this chapter, I was reminded of a conversation I recently had with two of my colleagues, John Miller and Edward Griffiths. We were delivering a leadership seminar to senior nurses and medical staff in Egypt for the Ministry of Health and Population and had included information and publications about Clinical Governance. However, in considering outcomes and expectations of healthcare, we all agreed that our own personal and professional experiences influence the view we have of healthcare provision. Like many of my nursing and midwifery colleagues, I am a person with a number of roles and experiences of our healthcare service. In my own case, it has encompassed being a professional, working as a clinician, educator, manager and researcher, but it has also encompassed being a patient and a patient's daughter, mother, wife and friend. For example, I experienced maternity services for the first time working as a student nurse 21 years ago, then as an expectant mother 14 years ago, and again as a later mother only two years ago. Like colleagues and patients, I have experienced first hand the dilemmas, the challenges and the improvements developing in healthcare.

In my professional life, when I specialized in oncology, we worked consistently to improve cancer services, to ensure that patients were treated as individuals, received quality information, had choice and were supported, to ensure that the physical and psychological assaults of disease and treatment were minimized, and to ensure that patients were treated by a specialist multidisciplinary team. These efforts were rewarded and what started as a mission of the few became an unstoppable movement. I would never claim that we have arrived, but there have been significant improvements in cancer care and as a result there are an army of professional and lay colleagues continuing to take the challenge forward.

In the field of quality, nurses and midwives have often led the way, working with patients and other professionals to deliver the highest possible standards of care. This commitment and valuable input to quality was highlighted in the nursing, midwifery and health visiting strategy document *Making a Difference*.[1] In my view, nurses and midwives are uniquely placed to deliver quality improvements where they are most needed – at the direct interface with the patient. There is no reason why this should change – certainly, the agenda has been refocused and an urgency brought to modernizing the Health Service, but the principles remain the same, namely to provide high-quality health care to patients that is responsive, provided equitably and is focused on the key issues facing our National Health Service (NHS).

Some nurses and midwives may have been given the impression that clinical governance is a medical preserve, but this is patently not the case – clinical governance is about patients. It is about providing quality services to patients in a spirit of true partnership – partnership between nurses, midwives, doctors and the multidisciplinary team, but more importantly between patients and the NHS. It is about creating a culture where true collaboration takes place and services are provided that meet patients' needs and expectations while at the same time allowing health professionals, including nurses and midwives, to deliver the best care of which they are capable. Clinical governance is

'a framework through which the NHS organisations are accountable for continuously improving the quality of their services and safeguarding high standards of care, by creating an environment in which excellence in clinical care will flourish.'

Explicit within this definition are what have been termed the seven pillars of establishing clear and effective patient and professional partnerships:

1. Clinical effectiveness
2. Risk management effectiveness
3. Patient experience
4. Communication effectiveness
5. Resource effectiveness
6. Strategic effectiveness
7. Learning effectiveness

It is also important to position such pillars upon firm foundations, which include systems awareness, teamwork, communication, ownership and leadership.

It is imperative that all professionals be engaged in this process. Nurses and midwives, in particular, have so much to contribute to the development of clinical governance, as they are so often at the forefront of quality innovation.

Nurses and midwives should be involved in setting up the framework for clinical governance in their particular clinical area. The scope of their responsibilities will obviously vary, depending on their role within the organization. Their organization will have set up lines of accountability and responsibility. Work should have been done to establish a baseline assessment and a development plan produced for taking the work forward.

Now that the Chief Executive has a statutory responsibility for the quality of care in an NHS provider, the focus on quality is acute. There should now be a culture where nurses' and midwives' concerns regarding the improvement of the quality of care for patients should be welcomed. The lead in day-to-day terms for the taking forward of clinical governance can be taken by a senior clinician, usually at board level. It could be a Medical Director, but now very frequently it is taken on by the Director of Nursing, often giving him or her the title Director of Nursing/Quality. Local commissioning groups are setting up their own arrangements for clinical governance, but again in a number of cases nurses and midwives are taking the lead, sometimes in cooperation with a GP.

The NHS provider's development plan is a fundamental document that nurses and midwives should participate actively in producing and monitoring. It is important that nurses and midwives at all levels know who is in the lead for clinical governance for their area.

It is important that nurses and midwives be aware and participate in the practical steps to ensure that clinical governance is a success. For nurses and midwives, there must be:

- A recognition that every member of staff in the multidisciplinary team has a unique role to play in the provision of high-quality care to their patients and clients.
- The understanding that clinical governance is about improving the quality of care using the most appropriate methods. The process involves identification of the problem, an assessment of the situation, a structured plan for improvement, monitoring of that plan, and evaluation of the outcome to ensure that future plans for improvement are informed by evidence.
- The understanding that clinical governance is about being accountable for your care to the wider world. Colleagues, patients and the public all want to be safe in the knowledge that they are receiving the most appropriate and skilful care possible.
- The understanding that the systems in which nurses and midwives work must be assessed to ensure that they are enabling them to work to the best of their ability. Poor physical conditions or poor organization can all impact on our ability to provide the best care of which we are capable.

Taking the elements of clinical governance into the practice environment, it is clear to see how our colleagues in practice have coordinated relevant functions to steer their thinking towards the achievement of quality care:

1. Standard setting
2. Clinical risk management
3. Use involvement
4. Clinical audit
5. Quality assurance
6. Evidence-based practice
7. Multidisciplinary working
8. Continuing education

Making up the essential elements or spokes of an inter-related wheel, it is evident how all contribute to the ultimate goal of working towards the achievement of quality care. To help in our understanding of contemporary practice, it is useful to consider case studies to help us focus upon changing practice.

Sister Ann Taylor had just taken up a new post in a major trauma Accident and Emergency Department. After working around the clock to get a feel for the department, she became conscious that although the numbers of nursing colleagues for staffing were adequate, she was aware of patients waiting for substantial periods to see the Senior House Officer at night. She noted the frustrations of patients and nursing staff who had to wait for a medical discharge even for minor injuries. These patients were often becoming irritated, and as a result a proportion of them were taking their own discharge against advice. Other patients with more complex injuries were often waiting longer than she felt acceptable, and once again the nursing staff felt powerless to improve the situation.

Ann was aware of the onus on her and all her colleagues to improve the situation, and as a result she had an informal conversation with the main A&E consultant Barbara Sims and made an appointment to come and discuss the situation further with her. Once they had shared their concerns together, Ann agreed to take the lead in conducting a baseline assessment to help them identify the strengths and weaknesses of the care they were providing. They agreed to share their thoughts and discussions at the multidisciplinary Team Meeting the following week.

The rest of the Team were feeling somewhat hesitant about the proposed exercise, but could see the potential value to the patients and to the rest of the staff. Ann and Barbara reassured them that once the baseline information was available, they would bring it back to the Team Meeting and share with them how the information related to their local Health Improvement Programmes and National Service Frameworks before they decided to go any further.

As Ann was in the lead for this initial assessment, she decided as part of the overall piece of work to conduct a SWOT analysis looking at the Department's

Strengths, Weaknesses, Opportunities and potential Threats. She asked as many of the staff who were willing to contribute their thoughts and observations, including the junior doctors, who felt, somewhat naturally, that they were being unjustly made the focus of attention.

Another approach that Ann adopted to get her baseline information was to conduct a significant-event audit. She chose this method because she felt it would be a reasonably straightforward way to look at a difficult situation. She brought together a cross-section of the staff and shared with them one of the incidents, which sparked her initial concerns.

At about 02:00, Ann had been doing her rounds in the department and had noticed a 70-year-old woman in one of the cubicles with her daughter beside her. The woman was a Mrs Davis, and it appeared that she had fallen down a flight of stairs just before midnight. After her fall, Mrs Davis managed to crawl to a telephone to ring her daughter, who came straight around and called an ambulance. The ambulance arrived at about 12:30 and Mrs Davis was admitted to the Department at about 01:00 with suspected head and/or neck fractures.

Mrs Davis was in obvious pain and acutely distressed at being secured in a neck and body brace. The department was reasonably busy, but there were adequate numbers of nursing staff present. The main limiting factor to Mrs Davis receiving prompt attention was the fact only one Casualty Officer was available at the time. Mrs Davis, who was in significant pain, was not seen by a doctor until 03:30. Mrs Davis and her daughter were polite, but it was obvious that they were not at all happy with the situation.

The nurses felt guilty and helpless, and as a result they did not go into the cubicle more often than was necessary. This avoidance on their part seemed to make the situation worse for them as well as for the patient and her daughter, who felt even more isolated.

Once Mrs Davis was seen by the SHO and a X-ray was requested, it was a further two hours before the results were conveyed to her, pain relief obtained and the brace removed. Mrs Davis had a fracture to her 4th cervical spine, but her head and upper neck were unaffected by the fall.

Mrs Davis was finally admitted to her ward at 08:00.

Ann asked the team to identify the key issues in this significant event. In their view, the key components were:

- medical staffing
- feelings of impotence due to role limitations
- pain control protocols
- communication and psychological support – provision for patients and staff

The team then discussed each area in turn, using the simple SWOT formula to creatively look at solutions for improving the care of other patients in a similar situation.

Once Ann had gathered the data and synthesized it, she and Barbara met to discuss the findings. They realized very quickly that there was an issue with medical staffing, which Barbara would pursue with the Medical Director, but there was also an issue about nursing and the very high level of education and skills that the nurses now possessed. Together, they agreed that Ann should discuss this with her Nurse Executive Director to discuss the options open to them to extend practice.

Ann and Barbara jointly shared the information gathered and outlined their suggestions for the next steps. The Team were interested but hesitant. The nursing staff could see the possibilities that a review might suggest, and became quite enthusiastic. The medical staff felt reassured that they were being offered support rather than criticism, but some of the support staff were concerned that any change might negatively impact on their workload.

The Team together decided that they would review the Trust's guidelines and take positive steps to generally take this work on quality, clinical governance, forward. They decided that they should look at a number of other areas, including:

- risk management
- developing information systems
- reviewing their medical audit procedures
- reviewing their nursing audit procedures
- reviewing their significant-event audit procedures
- strategic plans for professional development
- current objectives for the department

As a department, they realized someone would need to take the lead on implementing this new way of working and thinking in relation to clinical governance. One of the Lecturer Practitioners, Liz Hurley, felt that she would like to take the lead role as part of her ongoing professional development, provided that she had the full support of Ann and Barbara and the genuine cooperation of the rest of the staff.

Liz decided to identify and meet the Trust's lead person for clinical governance as well as seeking out other locally available sources of general information and support. She also decided to initiate meetings with other departments to identify their lead person for clinical governance to enable her to learn from their experiences so far.

Once the initial baseline assessment had been completed and the initial plans for action implemented, Ann was content that the Department was on its way to making a positive start. She and Barbara felt that the Department was committed to the clinical governance approach, and she felt sure that everyone realized their crucial contribution to making it happen.

The team agreed to work with Liz to ensure that their departmental priorities fitted into the Trust's priorities and was dovetailed into local priorities included in their local Health Improvement Programmes as well as national priorities such as the National Service frameworks.

As an A&E, they were aware that the national work on:

- antibiotic prescribing
- cancer services
- mental health services
- coronary heart disease

would obviously impact on them and the care they needed to provide to their patients.

As this case study has noted, nurses and midwives need to be aware of the sources of support and information available to them to enable them to fulfil their responsibilities – for example NHS guidelines, professional organization guidelines, clinical guidelines, systematic reviews and clinical research. There is also now an NHS Clinical Governance Support Team (CGST). As reported by the Department of Health, the CGST, through its innovative programmes, enables a wide variety of NHS organizations to involve staff and patients in improving services. Clinical governance, it is stated, is about changing the way in which people work, demonstrating that effective teamwork is as important to high-quality care as risk management and clinical effectiveness. The CGST has developed a number of development programmes that involve implementing clinical governance at a number of levels. The Team works directly with the NHS to support progress on clinical governance by empowering staff to make changes at a local level. Its work, which is profession-friendly and patient centred, serves to provide practical support through a helpline for NHS staff, through worked-up models of clinical governance in practice, and by focusing on leadership development. The Team is there to work with everyone, including nurses and midwives, to help us all overcome barriers to progress.

Having systems like those outlined is fundamental to enable us to create a healthcare system that is consistent and equitable, but to achieve this we must have the commitment of everyone working within an organization. Every nurse and midwife has a part to play, as part of an organization, as a professional and as an individual. As nurses and midwives, our role is different from that of a doctor or any other professional caring for patients. We are in the unique position of being well placed to influence colleagues and patients alike. We are clearly a professional group, which spans all healthcare environments from primary to acute care. We are already very comfortable with working within a multiagency environment. We have long promoted the concept of team working, but nurses and midwives need support too. It is vital that there is strong leadership in place, that continuing professional development is seen as vital and that appropriate information is continuously shared.

Good care depends on effective collaboration between many people. How those people work together is a crucial determinant of the quality of care. Within teams and when working on our own, nurses and midwives bring a unique contribution to the quality of care and more specifically to clinical governance. Nurses and midwives have a central place within any multidisciplinary team. They are often the only point of regular contact in a patient's care. Other professionals will become involved in a patient's care at different times, but quite often the nurse or midwife will be there throughout. This gives them a perspective that is invaluable. They can see where the interface between professionals and different organizations works well – and more importantly where it is not working well. Clinical governance spans the artificial barriers created by professions and organizations. It needs to follow the patients – to be patient-centred. Our insights need to be fed into the review of services, to ensure that change creates seamless care for the patient – whether they are receiving their care from nurses, midwives, doctors or therapists.

For example, Mr James is a 56-year-old professional man with chronic T-cell leukaemia. He is often neutropenic and anaemic. Mr James had been a chronic leukaemic for 12 years when he started to require blood transfusions every two weeks. During this period, he also started to pick up very severe infections, which could leave him unconscious very rapidly. Mr James's wife was obviously very frightened, but was reassured by the oncology team caring for him. Her main difficulty was the fact that she could not tell when he was becoming acutely ill, but because it all happened so quickly and as she couldn't drive, she was always in the position of having to call an ambulance. The ambulance would come and often some time would elapse before Mr James was admitted to the Oncology Ward with the nurses and doctors who knew him.

Staff Nurse Vince Hall realized the situation was causing Mr and Mrs James a great deal of concern and spoke to colleagues, who agreed with him that admission protocols needed updating, particularly for patients like Mr James. As a team, they did a piece of work looking at streamlining the service that chronic oncology patients experienced and set to work to ensure that everyone within and outside the department was aware of the new arrangements.

Vince discussed the new arrangements with Mr and Mrs James and ensured that their GP was content. In the future, all that Mrs James had to do was call an ambulance and let the ward know her husband was on his way in when she felt his condition was deteriorating. With the new system, admission formalities were bypassed until Mr James was safely on the ward, where immediate treatment and care could be started.

Nursing and midwifery professionals have always been at the forefront of involving patients and their carers in the planning and delivery of clinical care.

Their unique position can engender strong and trusting relationships with patients and families, and so create a unique opportunity to influence service provision so that it better meets patients' needs and expectations.

Nurses and midwives have often been involved in undertaking research to establish the views of patients and carers in many specialities. Research can focus on providing an evidence base not only to help us look for ways to improve care but also to identify problems. In our illustration, Ann chose to use a significant-event audit as a tool in gathering her baseline information, but other options are possible. Problems can be identified by:

- encouraging free and open communication
- providing staff with supportive clinical supervision
- conducting a needs assessment
- monitoring all letters of complaint or praise regularly and looking out for recurring themes or issues
- surveying patients
- using quality published research to compare the results or recommendations with current practice
- conducting a formal research study subject to scientific and ethics committee approval

At one time, it was very easy to see a patient as a series of symptoms – a puzzle to be solved, an illness to be cured. But patients are more than that, and nurses and midwives are very good at seeing patients as human beings who need both care and cure (if possible). This care may be much wider than the direct treatment of a set of symptoms. This perspective and a focus on caring is, I believe, a fundamental strength of nurses, midwives and health visitors. We need to see beyond the symptoms to the patient and work to provide care to them in a comprehensive and cohesive way. There is no point in X-raying an elderly woman for a fracture, reassuring her that all is well, and then discharging her in the middle of the night to an empty flat.

Throughout the country, health visitors, while encouraging and enabling young families to make full use of developmental and health screening services, also concentrate on helping young people to become confident parents by teaching them parenting skills and putting them in touch with voluntary and statutory organizations. They may, for example, need help in accessing Social Services in sorting out a housing problem, or they may need to be introduced to the school nurse, who will be able to assist the older child who has been having problems settling into his new class. By taking this holistic approach, health visitors are stretching their role and therefore their accountability, which requires them at all times to be fully aware of their responsibilities within set regulations.

Evaluation of nurse-led services demonstrates that because nurses are in contact longer with the patient than doctors are, they are able to discuss more fully the range of options open to patients. Advising patients and their families is an increasingly important part of the professional role, making sound, evidence-based information available to them and actively supporting their choices so that the patients themselves are participants in, not merely recipients of, healthcare. Information and information technology are valuable assets in this process.

The nursing and midwifery professions regularly use operational clinical systems to extract and analyse information – for example:

- to identify patients suffering from a particular condition or to measure the incidence of pressure sores
- to assess compliance with treatment protocols in line with National Service Frameworks
- to check compliance with monitoring processes to manage and avoid long-term complications
- to monitor outcomes of care

– and an increasingly wide range of material will become available, for example, through the NHS Net and the Electronic Library for Health.

Nurses must use evidence-based information to inform their practice, and to communicate information to their patients so that they are actively engaged in decisions about their healthcare.

As medicine has advanced, many of the treatments offered to patients have become more and more complex. It is easy in such areas to lose sight of what the care is intended to do – to improve the health of the patient. In many cases, treatment has grown incrementally as time has gone by and new ways of delivering elements of care have been developed. Often there is a need to step back from the detail and look at the big picture. We need to ensure that the appropriate professional delivers services in the most clinically effective way, in the most suitable setting. Because nurses and midwives are in contact with patients for prolonged periods of time, they are able to tease out the likely concerns that patients have and ensure that services are developed in such a way as to reflect their individual needs.

Benchmarking techniques are increasingly being used by groups of practitioners to structure the comparison and sharing of examples of good practice to address patients' concerns about the quality of nursing care, such as complaints about not being washed, not being fed, not being treated with respect, etc. Benchmarks of best practice are identified by patients and professionals as a means of identifying the essential elements of high-quality care, and this provides important information on which to establish an improvement-based approach to clinical practice and service delivery. The NHS Executive is establishing regional support networks for clinical benchmarking activity. Regional facilitators will assist in establishing comparison groups of practitioners, who can then use the benchmarks to pull together to identify action plans that will ensure that practice is shared and developed to consistently achieve high-quality care.

We have considered some of the ways in which nurses and midwives can contribute to the clinical governance agenda. Clinical governance will lead to exciting changes in the ways in which services are delivered. The role of nurses and midwives is changing and we need to ensure that this continues to enable the new challenges ahead to be met. We are already beginning to see this happening in many of the key initiatives within the NHS. In the document *Liberating the Talents. Helping Primary Care Trusts and Nurses to Deliver the NHS Plan*,[2] John Hutton (Minister of Health, 2002) stated that 90% of all patients' journeys begin and end in primary care. Liberating the talents provides primary care organizations and front-line staff with a new framework for planning and delivering nursing services in primary care, by providing a coherent strategic direction and practical support for change.

But other new and now established roles have proved to be important in moving the NHS forward, while also establishing and moulding nursing and midwifery within responsive and flexible frameworks to meet an ever-changing society.

NHS Direct

NHS Direct, the nurse-led service, puts nursing firmly at the forefront of the drive to develop more accessible and responsive healthcare. It aims to provide prompt access to professional advice and reassurance 24 hours a day, 365 days a year. It can enable patients to care for themselves at home or directs them quickly to the right service, at the right time. NHS Direct aims to empower patients to take greater control of their own health and well-being.

It is clearly an innovation that works to benefit patients, but it also opens exciting and challenging opportunities for nurses – opportunities to make better use of their knowledge and skills and to build on these skills in a dynamic environment, as well as opportunities to take the lead in developing a service that provides the very best of care and support to patients and their families.

NHS Direct is an example of how nursing professionals can make a difference by working in partnership with patients.

Walk-in Centres

Walk-in Centres – all of which are nurse-led – provide another unique opportunity. The services provided by these Centres aim to enable the public to make informed choices about their own health and to encourage them to use services in the appropriate way. Centres will provide a range of services, including advice about self-care, healthy lifestyles, and management of minor ailments and injuries. They will also direct people to other health services – both statutory and voluntary – often in conjunction with NHS Direct. They should be conveniently located and open at times that suit modern lifestyles. They are intended to compliment existing Primary Care Centres.

Nurses and midwives will need to work flexibly and will need to be adaptable in order to respond appropriately to user requirements. We will need to continue to recognize the importance of diversity and the need to respect the right of users to exercise their choice. In particular, we will have to ensure that the information that we provide is up-to-date and communicated in a responsible, relevant and timely way.

The role that Walk-in Centres will play in other new initiatives is also becoming well acknowledged, such as the *Out-of-Hours Review*, which has put forward a flexible integrated model of out-of-hours GP provision.[3]

It is also important to reflect upon the emerging Emergency Care Practitioner (ECP), with the recent publication by the NHS Modernisation Agency of the *Emergency Care Practitioner Review – Right Skill, Right Time, Right Place*.[4] This report illustrates the development of the ECP's role in the management of patients who require emergency (unscheduled) care. It raises awareness of the ECP's role and its potential impact on the whole system of unscheduled-care reform. The report refers to current practices that can be adopted/adapted locally with regard to the development of the ECP.

New roles for nurses in primary care

Taking cognisance of the document *Liberating the Talents. Helping Primary Care Trusts and Nurses to deliver the NHS Plan*[2] and its provision of a new framework for planning and delivering nursing services in primary care, by providing a coherent strategic direction and practical support for change, it is worth remembering that within the primary care agenda, nurses are now considering new and influential roles.

At a clinical level, nurse prescribing has offered the opportunity for over 25 000 nurses with a district nursing or health visiting qualification to be trained to prescribe.

Throughout the country, practice nurses are now essential members of Primary Care Teams, leading the way in running clinics and in providing expert support to patients and expert advice to professional colleagues.

For patients, nurse involvement in key roles in primary care and in building integrated care pathways provides a more consistent and effective approach to healthcare delivery – one that works and one that patients trust.

From the nurses' perspective, it enhances our role, giving us opportunities to take on new responsibilities and to be truly accountable for the quality of service provided.

Nurse Consultants

Nurse Consultants are now a reality, and working at this level will be a challenge to the post-holders to be able to synthesize, coherently and effectively, knowledge and expertise related to an area of practice. They will need to apply new knowledge to their own and others' practice in structured ways that can be evaluated, as well as interpreting and evaluating information from diverse sources to make informed judgements about its quality and appropriateness.

Nurse Consultants have the opportunity to actively monitor the effectiveness of current therapeutic programmes and integrate different aspects of practice to improve outcomes for patients and clients, while managing constantly changing scenarios in the interest of patients and clients.

Key to their role is the promotion of the improvement of quality and clinical effectiveness within resource constraints. In order to do this, they will have to continuously assess and monitor risk in their own and others' practice, as well as challenging others about wider risk factors.

An essential element of the ability of Nurse Consultants to achieve what has just been described will be their ability to continually evaluate and audit their own practice and that of others. This involves applying a broad range of valid and reliable evaluation methods, as well as utilizing critical appraisal skills to synthesize the outcomes of research evaluations and audits and apply them to improve practice.

Whichever way we look, nurses and midwives are demonstrating their wide-ranging ability to be full members of the healthcare team taking clinical governance forward in partnership with patients and clients. The undoubted expertise that nurses and midwives possess will help to improve services. As nurses and midwives, we must consistently build on current excellence, as well as constantly identifying and rectifying poorer performance as part of our corporate responsibility within our organizations. Nurses and midwives have a significant contribution to make to the clinical governance agenda, and I am confident that we will be seen to be making it.

The views expressed in this chapter are personal, and all names in the case studies are fictitious.

References

1. *Making a Difference. Strengthening the Nursing, Midwifery and Health Visiting Contribution to Health and Healthcare.* London: Department of Health, 1999.
2. *Liberating the Talents. Helping Primary Care Trusts and Nurses to Deliver the NHS Plan.* London: Department of Health, 2004.
3. *Implementing the Out of Hours Review.* London: Department of Health, 2004.
4. *The Emergency Care Practitioner – Right Skill, Right Time, Right Place.* London: Department of Health, 2004.
5. *A First Class Service: Quality in the New NHS.* London: Department of Health, 1998.
6. Roland M, Baker R. *Clinical Governance: A Practical Guide for Primary Care Teams.* Manchester: University of Manchester, 1999.
7. *Clinical Governance: How Nurses Can Get Involved.* London: Royal College of Nursing, 2000.

8	The role of the medical director in ensuring high-quality care
	Rowland B Hopkinson

Introduction

The medical director in the UK, whether working in acute, mental health or primary care settings, has a fundamental role to play in establishing services that provide high-quality patient care. Unfortunately, these aims can be frustrated by the difficulties of providing a contracted level of activity for a given financial resource. Given these conflicting demands, service quality issues may not receive the priority that they deserve despite the earnest desire of medical directors for higher standards. The current and desired positions are illustrated by the Venn diagrams is Figure 8.1(a) and (b) respectively.

In (a), which typifies the situation in the National Health Service (NHS) in 2004, financial returns are a consequence of activity and quality of care is largely irrelevant as a primary focus of interest. The 'high-quality' vision (b)

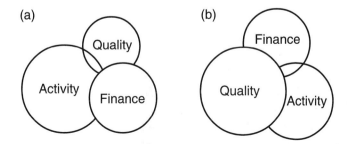

FIGURE 8.1 (a) Current and (b) desired service quality positions.

has to be of investment in quality, enabling efficient and effective activity, which in turn provides the financial return. This requires care providers (Trusts) and commissioners to take the highly challenging step of relying upon investment in improving the quality of service (change), delivering economic and activity benefit; perhaps this might also be a consequence of giving patients a genuine choice as to where they are treated.

It is the aim of this chapter to demonstrate the levers that are available to medical directors to help them provide a high-quality service despite financial and activity pressures. These levers for high-quality come in the form of the need for the Trust Boards of Directors to be provided with assurance about the services that the organization delivers and also to respond to centrally set standards that the NHS and the public require. While these issues are discussed in the context of the NHS in England, the principles are equally applicable in other settings. Indeed, it can be argued that the quality of systems in England lags behind those of some other home nations.

Structures available to drive the improvement of quality

Clinical governance

Scally and Donaldson[1] originally propounded clinical governance in 1998. The Government's White Paper, *A First Class Service*, defined clinical governance as:

> 'a framework through which NHS organizations are accountable for continuously improving the quality of their services and safeguarding high standards of care by creating an environment in which excellence in clinical care will flourish.'

It created a statutory duty for improving quality through a process of setting, delivering and monitoring standards of care, underpinned by a culture of lifelong learning and professional self-regulation.

As clinical governance has evolved since 1998, its various components have been identified; all are relevant to the role of the medical director. These can be summarized as:

- ensuring that clinical governance principles, processes and systems are embedded at the trust board and within the organization

- ensuring that at a local level there are systems in place to ensure the delivery of safe, high-quality care
- ensuring the implementation of the national quality initiatives, e.g. National Patient Safety Agency (NPSA) reporting, National Institute for Clinical Excellence (NICE) guidance and National Service Framework (NSF) standards
- ensuring participation in national confidential enquiries
- ensuring that all clinicians are involved in regular clinical audit and review of clinical services
- assessing performance and identifying training needs for all staff
- developing an open culture within the organization where incidents are reported and lessons are learned
- ensuring that effective risk management processes are in place
- monitoring trends in clinical quality and clinical outcome
- maintaining a focus on continuous, demonstrable improvement in the quality of the patient experience and of healthcare outcomes
- involving partners in service provision in clinical governance activities
- assuming and making clear the joint accountability for services that are provided on a multi-agency, multisector basis
- reporting to Strategic Health Authorities on clinical governance activities

Controls assurance

As clinical governance developed, the Government recognized a need for assurance that high-quality patient care was delivered in organizations operating within a system of internal control. It is a process designed to provide evidence that NHS organizations are doing their reasonable best to manage themselves so as to meet their objectives and protect patients, staff, the public and other stakeholders against risks of all kinds.[2]

This resulted in the development of the controls assurance programme. It sets out a rigorous programme of control standards across more than 20 areas within every NHS organization and covers clinical and non-clinical functions. The standards require very detailed and specific actions of organizations to assure the Trust Board and Government that systems of internal control exist. Table 8.1 demonstrates their wide area of influence and also the fact that many are of relevance clinically and hence a concern for medical directors.

Over the past three years, the Government has worked towards the convergence of the clinical governance and controls assurance agendas. This is reflected in the discussions that follow.

TABLE 8.1 Controls assurance standards

- Buildings, land, plant and non-medical equipment standard
- Catering and food hygiene
- Decontamination of medical devices
- Emergency planning
- Environmental management
- Financial management (core standard)
- Fire safety
- Governance (core standard)
- Health and safety
- Human resources
- Infection control
- Information management and technology
- Managing of purchasing and supply
- Medical equipment and devices
- Medicines management
- Professional advice and services
- Records management
- Risk management system (core standard)
- Security management
- Fleet and transport management
- Waste management
- Research governance standard

Inter-related strategies

There are also a whole series of other strategies that have a significant impact upon the healthcare industry in the UK. They must therefore be considered (and used) by medical directors as a part of any scheme to improve the quality of care. Strategies/initiatives to be considered include:

- The NHS Plan
- Patient and Public Involvement
- Improving Working Lives
- Agenda for Change
- Clinical Governance Reviews – Healthcare Commission/CHI
- Performance Star Ratings
- First Class Service
- Organisation with a Memory
- Building a Safer NHS for Patients
- National Patient Safety Agency
- NHS Litigation Authority

- Payment by results
- Choose and Book

Board assurance

Every year, Chief Executives of NHS Trusts, on behalf of their Boards, have to sign a *Statement of Internal Control*. This forms part of the statutory accounts and annual report. Trust Boards need to be able to demonstrate that they had been properly informed through assurances about the totality of risk in their organization (not just financial) and have arrived at their conclusions based on all the evidence presented to them.

Published by the Department of Health, *Assurance – the Board Agenda*[3] explains how this should be done. It sets the parameters by which the provider Board can assure itself that the systems and processes established within trust are safe and effective. The circular states that Boards can only properly fulfil their responsibilities if they have a sound understanding of the principal risks facing the organization. They then have to determine the assurance that they require with regard to those risks.

Each trust should have designed its own framework for understanding the principal risks that the organization faces. In turn, Board-level objectives should reflect the management of these risks. This will take place as the Board debates and maps the connections linking organizational objectives, risk, and the range and effectiveness of reporting. The Board and the organization have to decide what is *reasonable* rather than expecting absolute assurance.

While some of the substantial risks will undoubtedly be financial, there will be those associated with attaining high clinical standards, management of staff and ensuring the efficient use of resources.

The medical director has a vital role to play in this process, particularly in contributing to the understanding of non-executive directors about clinical standards in the organization. Through this route, medical directors have an opportunity to exercise substantial influence to improve the quality of care given by the organization. They will, with other senior managers and staff, help the Board to determine the significance of risks, taking into account existing and planned management assurance and action, as well as any mitigating factors. In essence, the Trust constructs a high-level risk register.

Audit

Assurance for the Board, about risks and the quality of care, will also be provided from a number of sources, including external and internal auditors, other external assessors such as the Clinical Negligence Scheme for Trusts (CNST), and now the Healthcare Commission. The medical director can use these audits to identify or highlight important clinical issues. Indeed, it is important that the focus of Trust audit committees be given a wider perspective than just financial matters.

Medical directors must be involved in these Trust activities and should not allow them, and their influence, to be dominated by financial and/or activity issues. It is to be hoped that in the future the scope and interest of audit committees extend further into clinical areas.

However, the drive for Foundation Trust status places, necessarily, even greater emphasis on business and financial functions. Monitor (the independent regulator for Foundation Trusts) has relatively little interest in clinical issues.[4] As a minimum, medical directors should involve themselves in the conduct of value-for-money (VFM) audits and their use as a quality improvement tool.

External quality controls

In July 2004, the Department of Health published a document entitled *National Standards, Local Action*. With it was published *Standards for Better Health*.[5] The standards described the level of quality that all healthcare organizations will be expected to provide for NHS patients. The standards integrate a previously disparate group of quality parameters in terms of–

1. safety
2. clinical and cost-effectiveness
3. governance
4. patient focus
5. accessible and responsive care
6. care environment and amenities
7. public health

Each of these domains has *core standards*, which bring together and rationalize existing requirements. There are also *developmental standards*, which signal a direction of travel for the improvement of services. NSFs and NICE guidance are integral to this standards-based system.

These standards will provide a framework for NHS bodies to plan the delivery of services, and their improvement, in line with increasing patient, public, political and media expectations. They will also form a key part of the performance assessment of organizations by the Healthcare Commission, which will be applying them in this context.

For medical directors in Wales, the Advisory Board for Healthcare Standards in Wales has published its own consultation document.[6] This provides a somewhat different structure, using four domains:

- the patient experience
- clinical outcomes
- healthcare governance
- public health

Patient focus and safety issues are addressed within these four domains rather than separately. Certainly, as far as patient safety is concerned, there is undoubted merit in this approach as, from a clinical perspective, management of risk is a vital component of all clinical care.

Until detailed assessment criteria are applied to these high-level standards, it will be difficult to be sure whether the same can be said of accessibility, important as it is. In Wales, the application of the standards will be reviewed by the Healthcare Inspectorate Wales (HIW). As in England, medical directors need to be aware of these developments, as these standards can be used very effectively to improve patient care.

The Government and the Healthcare Commission say that organizations will be assessed on reduced numbers of national targets as well as on whether they are delivering high-quality care against these standards. New targets will be about health outcomes and patient experience.

The document also lays emphasis on the benefits that can accrue from implementation of the National Programme for Information Technology (NPfIT). The hope is that making better use of staff time, service redesign and workforce reform will also improve standards.

In all these aspects, the medical director has a crucial role to play, particularly in ensuring that old-fashioned clinical practices are not perpetuated in changed systems. New systems must be used to support changes in service delivery that have a clear patient focus.

All of this develops the theme of clinical governance. Medical directors should note that the Department of Health now has a series of definitions:

- *standards* are a means of describing the level of quality that healthcare organizations are expected to meet or aspire to, and which enable their performance to be assessed
- *quality requirements* describe the care that clinicians will use to guide their practice (e.g. through NSFs)
- *criteria* are ways of demonstrating compliance with, and performance relevant to, a standard.
- *targets* are referred to in order to define the level of performance
- *benchmarks* are used as comparators for comparing similar organizations

Core standards

Core standards are based on requirements that already exist within the NHS. These are not optional, describing the level of service that is only acceptable but that must be universal. Medical directors should already be applying them in their organizations.

Developmental standards

These are to provide a focus for the health service to improve over time. Criteria are to be developed against which progress can be measured.

Given the influential position of medical directors or equivalents within healthcare systems, it is inevitable that they will have a significant role in implementing such standards. Again, these standards give them the levers to significantly improve the quality of care delivered within their organization.

The domains described in the standards documentation provide a useful vehicle to explore the opportunities and responsibilities of medical directors in improving services.

First domain: safety

Ensuring that patients come to as little harm as possible is a fundamental role for the medical director. Participation in activities that reduce risk is an essential component of providing a high-quality service. This core standard requires that organizations identify and learn from all patient safety incidents, including safety notices and alerts from other organizations such as the NPSA.

The standard also requires organizations to take steps to protect children, follow NICE interventional procedures guidance, reduce healthcare-acquired infection, use medicines securely and safely, and also minimize the risks to the health and safety of staff, patients and the public.

How can this be applied in practice? What is the role of the medical director?

The medical director must ensure that the Trust has in place governance structures that can deal with all these issues. It is unlikely that they will be able to participate personally in all aspects of clinical risk management, but they must be assured that a system exists for dealing with internal and external demands.

Claims, complaints and incidents – a virtuous cycle

Within the Trust's healthcare governance structure, there should be a clinical risk manager responsible dealing with claims, complaints and incidents, both trivial and serious. In large Trusts, there are likely to be hundreds of complaints each year and thousands of incidents reported. The medical director must ensure that there are mechanisms in place to classify complaints and incidents, identify important trends, report these trends into the operational machinery and ensure that action plans are developed to minimize future occurrence. The risk management governance structure will also need to be able to demonstrate that action plans have been implemented. This virtuous cycle of learning for staff working with patients is the most difficult for medical directors to establish. The contribution of doctors to clinical incident reporting has to be regarded as positive in the appraisal process, and any failure to contribute should call for discussion and potential criticism.

Medical directors need to be directly involved in the management of serious incidents, serious complaints and claims. Not only will they need to advise on the clinical significance of what is taking place, but they should also provide a commentary on the root-cause analysis that must be done to identify any underlying faults in systems and processes throughout the Trust.

When dealing with medico-legal claims, Trust solicitors will often provide summaries that include risk management issues that the operational organization needs to address. Again, the medical director must ensure that there are mechanisms in place for clinical areas to provide action plans that address these issues and that these action plans are implemented. This monitoring should take place in regular clinical governance meetings within the relevant clinical area and should be reported, by exception, to the subcommittee of the Trust Board responsible for clinical governance activities.

The incentives to do this are substantial because there is the opportunity not only to improve clinical care but also to prevent claims and reduce the costs of litigation.

For acute Trusts with large obstetric departments, the contingency costs for litigation will run into tens of millions of pounds, of which two-thirds will be for obstetrics. Investing time and effort in implementing risk management methodologies should stem the increase in costs of claims and hopefully reduce the escalation in the number of claims in an increasingly litigious society.

By implementing such systems, Trusts can also reduce the subscription that they pay to the NHS Litigation Authority through the Clinical Negligence Scheme for Trusts (CNST). For acute trusts – again particularly those with large obstetric units – the subscription can be several million pounds each year. The discounts available for obtaining CNST are substantial and illustrated in Table 8.2. The discounts can be invested to improve the quality of patient care and to fund governance mechanisms.

TABLE 8.2 CNST discounts

Level 1: 10% discount
Level 2: 20% discount
Level 3: 30% discount

External risk reporting arrangements

Within the governance arrangements of Trusts, there must be mechanisms for receiving reports for external agencies (such as the NPSA and the Chief Medical Officer) and disseminating them. There must also be mechanisms for reporting back. Currently, serious untoward incidents (SUIs) have to be reported to the NPSA and Strategic Health Authorities. If there is the potential for litigation, the NHSLA and the Trust solicitors may also have to be consulted.

All may have to be involved when the coroner investigates cases. The management of such issues can take a considerable amount of a medical director's time but is generally worth the investment. Good relationships and close liaison with Trust solicitors can save time and enable staff to be supported appropriately in what is becoming an increasingly hostile environment. The key is that medical directors ensure that lessons are learnt and disseminated.

Control of infection

Over the past two years, control of infection has become not only an increasing clinical worry but also an area of considerable public and media concern. While MRSA (methicillin-resistant *Staphylococcus aureus*) receives the attention of the media, other resistant bacteria and viral infections should be of equal concern for both staff and patients.

It is the medical director's responsibility to ensure that there are appropriate mechanisms in place for monitoring the incidence of colonization, infection and outbreaks. The medical director must also ensure that training is in place for all relevant staff in basic hygiene procedures, that appropriate records be kept of the training, that it be reinforced at agreed intervals and that the application of the training be audited regularly (e.g. handwashing).

With the chief executive of the Trust, the medical director will want to ensure that there is a properly constituted control of infection committee and a director of infection prevention and control. It is essential that sufficient resource be provided for infection control management and training.

There are a number of other areas of risk management that medical directors should ensure are heard within the organization, particularly by clinicians. There should be a transfusion committee to deal with blood transfusion problems and to consider serious hazards of transfusion (SHoT) issues. It is important to ensure that reporting back takes place. Resuscitation must also be properly organized, with appropriate audit so that the organization knows its failure rate. Health and safety issues are not highly regarded by clinicians; however, with the increasingly proactive approach by the Health and Safety Executive, this must change. Management of sharps injuries, stress, and violence and aggression are areas of concern within the health service.

There should also be clear lines of reporting of issues about prescribing, as medication errors cause significant problems in the health service.

Second domain: clinical and cost-effectiveness

This standard specifies that patients should benefit from decisions based upon assessed research evidence. The standard requires that:

- Healthcare organizations must conform to NICE technology appraisals and take into account nationally agreed guidance (e.g. NSFs).
- Care must be delivered in a well-led and supervised environment.
- Clinicians working in this environment must demonstrate that they continually update their skills and participate in regular clinical audit and the review of their clinical services.

The developmental standards extend these principles to ensure that patients' holistic needs are met and that a seamless service is developed, not just within the health service but within social care as well.

It is essential that the medical director ensure that there are systems in place within the organization, not only to react to external guidance but also to horizon-scan to identify new initiatives early in their 'life cycle'. The systems will quite logically parallel those for risk management within the healthcare governance structure.

Again, it is important that this activity, while being managed at the top of the organization, is embedded in the clinical areas, with clear lines of reporting that can provide the Trust Board with the necessary assurances that patients within the organization are being treated in the most up-to-date way. At the same term, the introduction of new procedures and innovative treatments must be regulated to ensure not only that the staff delivering them are appropriately trained, but also that patients are led to understand the risks.

As clinicians develop and update their skills, comprehensive records need to be retained by the organization to demonstrate their competency. The medical director also needs to ensure that all clinicians participate in useful, regular and systematic audit.

It is essential that medical directors ensure that their organizations provide sufficient support to facilitate this activity. It is no longer something that can be left to part-time enthusiasts. It must be made comprehensive and systematic if it is to deliver fundamental improvements in the quality of care provided.

Third domain: governance

The outcome required here is that managerial and clinical leadership and accountability ensure that probity, quality assurance, quality improvement and patient safety are central components of all the activities of the organization.

The core standards within the domain require healthcare organizations to actively support, among other requirements, a culture of openness, honesty, probity and accountability. There needs to be systematic risk assessment and risk management while ensuring that financial management achieves economy, effectiveness and efficiency.

To do this, healthcare organizations have to establish processes that enable staff to raise, in confidence and without prejudicing their position, concerns over any aspect of service delivery, treatment or management that they consider to have had a detrimental effect on patient care.

To this end, organizations are required to have a systematic and planned approach to the management of records. They also need to ensure that their employees have appropriate professional qualifications, are registered with the appropriate bodies and abide by any relevant codes of professional practice.

All staff are required to participate in relevant mandatory training programmes (including induction) and to have further professional development throughout their careers.

The developmental standards extend these requirements to the underpinning of the work of every clinical team, with a cycle of continuous quality improvement, under an umbrella of effective clinical and managerial leadership.

Professional codes of conduct

For the medical director, these standards provide an even greater challenge. In the clinical community, probity (or a lack of it) has not been regarded as a substantial issue. However, doctors will be increasingly tested upon the substance of their contribution to the NHS, their dealings with the private sector and with drug companies. Medical directors have to ensure that professional codes of conduct (notably the General Medical Council's *Good*

Medical Practice for doctors) are understood and implemented. As directors of an organization, they have shared responsibility for the application of codes of conduct for other staff groups. Here, they will work closely with and support the nursing director and the director of human resources.

Staff personal development

Medical directors have to ensure that there are systems of appraisal in place that test the compliance of clinicians with these codes of conduct; this is particularly important for doctors, as it is likely in the future to become part of the revalidation process.

Not only must the systems for appraisal be in place, but supporting training programmes must be there as well. All members of the clinical team must be able to demonstrate that they have attended mandatory and statutory training. It is no longer acceptable for groups of employees, notably doctors, to evade the requirement for them to undertake induction, fire training, manual handling and other instruction. Medical directors have a responsibility to ensure that such programmes are available, that they are attended and that a formal record is retained within the organization of such training. Demonstration that clinical staff have the necessary competencies is a requirement of CNST.

For all clinicians, appraisal should lead to a personal development plan. For new entrants into the organization, participation in a mentoring programme will provide support for a new role in a potentially unfamiliar environment. Medical directors need to ensure that there exists a cadre of suitably trained mentors to meet this requirement.

They will also need to consider whether other support, such as coaching, may be appropriate for more established senior clinicians. This can be provided for individuals or teams.

Fourth domain: patient focus

The stated outcome of this domain is that healthcare is provided in partnership with patients, their carers and with other organizations, such as social services, whose services affect patient well being.

The core standards refer to the treatment of patients with dignity and respect, the obtaining of appropriate consent, the confidential use of information, the provision of a complaints process that is responsive and promotes change, and the supply of information to patients about the clinical care that they receive.

Consent and patient information

This latter supply of information is essential for patients to make an informed choice about the treatment that they require and to provide valid consent. Medical directors need to ensure that the Department of Health instructions on consent can be shown to be in use throughout the organization and that this consent is supported by clear information that supplies patients with data on outcomes from procedures. This can either be done locally or else from a number of commercial websites; however, the Department of Health has also published proposals for a national system.[7]

Information governance and confidentiality

In many organizations, the medical director will also be the Caldicott Guardian, responsible for preventing inappropriate distribution of patient information. This enforcement of the Data Protection Act has become a complex responsibility, with numbers of stakeholders (e.g. Primary Care Trusts and Cancer Networks) expecting access to un-anonymized information.

The implementation of information governance standards and scoring, using the toolkit devised by the NHS Information Authority, means that this is rapidly moving beyond the capacity of individual medical directors. They are going to have to ensure that their healthcare governance structure has in it an individual with prime responsibility for implementation of these standards, who may then report to the medical director.

Medical records

It is also a requirement of CNST that medical staff not only complete the medical record but also clearly identify themselves. Medical directors need to ensure that audits are conducted to demonstrate that appropriate standards of record keeping are maintained and especially that medical staff can be identified.

Fifth domain: accessible and responsive care

The outcome measured in this domain is that patients should receive services as promptly as possible, have choice in access to services and do not experience unnecessary delays through the care pathway.

The core standards require that the views of patients and their carers be sought and taken into account in designing, planning, delivering and improving healthcare services. There should also be equity of access for emergency and elective care within nationally agreed timescales.

The developmental standards require healthcare organizations to provide services based on nationally agreed evidence and best practice in an environment that maximizes patient choice.

Medical directors clearly have an important role to play in ensuring that the services in their organizations meet these standards. They must promote an understanding of patients' views while, at the same time, interpreting for them their responsibilities and the realities of care. Medical directors must also try to ensure that patients' representatives and local politicians advertise the responsibility of individuals to use the healthcare system appropriately.

Sixth domain: care environment and amenities

Here the need to provide an environment that promotes patient and staff well-being is emphasized. Facilities must be provided for the effective and safe delivery of treatment, giving as much privacy as possible, in buildings that are clean and well maintained. The developmental standards lay emphasis on effective control of healthcare-associated infection.

Medical directors will support the standards with enthusiasm. They can be used to lever the provision of modern facilities that can enhance the morale of staff and patients. New premises can also enable the reduction of cross-infection and resulting patient morbidity.

To succeed here, medical directors must contribute to plans for site development and intervene if it appears that proposed facilities will not meet these requirements. For a secondary care service that has been primarily based upon communal wards, this means radical change in requiring a significant increase in the provision of individual rooms; just as in the UK's private sector.

A prerequisite for such delivery has to be an increase in nurse staffing, particularly if, as has been suggested, 50% of beds are to be provided in cubicles.

Medical directors must also be aware of the backlog maintenance requirements within their organizations and what new equipment is likely to be required, so that they can drive appropriate replacement programmes.

Seventh domain: public health

The essence of the proposals in this domain relates to the development of strategic partnerships involving directors of public health and local authorities in the development of managed disease prevention and health promotion programmes. These are particularly directed at obesity, smoking, substance misuse and sexually transmitted infections. The standard also identifies requirements to have plans to cope with major incidents and other emergency situations.

Medical directors have responsibility for ensuring that these latter plans are in place and practised regularly, in concert with other emergency services. They must also be involved in the development of services for chronic disease management, which will increasingly involve patient management in the community and less so in secondary care hospitals. Medical directors of acute Trusts and primary care services will have to work together to manage this interface, with a resulting reduction in the need for acute beds but with an increasing level of dependency in those that remain.

The Healthcare Commission will, in England, assess this intimidating array of standards.

Healthcare Commission: assessment for improvement[8]

The rapidity with which accreditation processors are being developed in the UK has been demonstrated by the publication of this document, which enlarges upon the standards and proposes guiding principles for a new approach to assessing performance. The guiding principles are shown in Table 8.3.

TABLE 8.3 Healthcare Commission – principles of assessment

1. Promote improvement and focus on outcomes
2. Take the perspective of the public and patients
3. Emphasize that healthcare organizations must assure themselves of the quality of their organization. Trust boards will need to assure themselves that they meet the core standards
4. Measure what matters for users, recognizing the different types of healthcare organizations. The ambition of the Healthcare Commission is to provide a rounded view of performance in all sectors
5. Use information intelligently. Emphasis here is on collection of information that is useful to patients, the public and providers of healthcare
6. Assess performance, not managed performance
7. Work in partnership with other regulators. In June 2004, 10 bodies concerned with inspection, regulation and audits published a *concordat* aiming to improve the quality and coordination of inspection while reducing the burden upon organizations
8. Target our work, allowing healthcare staff to do their work
9. Ensure that our people do the right things in the right place
10. Deliver robust judgements through open and fair processes
11. Ensure that our process of assessment provides value for money

The theme is to use inspection only when organizations have not demonstrated consistently good performance. Local intelligence and information will be used rather than formal visits and inspections, and evidence should only come from existing sources.

Medical directors will greet these suggestions with enthusiasm, and there will be relief that some rationalization of the processes of inspection is envisaged. However, in practice, existing targets are expected to be met through to 2007 (Tables 8.4 and 8.5). There are, however, new standards, and it is unlikely that those existing currently will remain unaltered given the current political desire to force change in the service (Table 8.6).

The Healthcare Commission will identify:

- the measurable elements of the standards
- the key issues or *prompts* that trusts may wish to consider in satisfying themselves that they meet core standards
- the most relevant indicators to be used for initial checks on performance and outcomes of each core standard

Having issued guidance on the core standards, the Healthcare Commission will then seek a declaration from both the Trust and its local partners as to how far they have complied with the standards. The Commission will then seek corroboration of the results that the Trust has achieved and institute spot checks if they have concerns and also of a random number of organizations. There will then be reporting and follow up.

TABLE 8.4 Commitments due to be achieved before March 2005[a]

- Reduce to 4 hours the maximum wait in A&E from arrival to admission, transfer or discharge
- Guarantee access to a primary care professional within 24 hours and to a primary care doctor within 48 hours
- All ambulance trusts to respond to 75% of Category A calls within 8 minutes
- All ambulance trusts to respond to 95% of category A calls within 14(urban)/19(rural) minutes
- All ambulance trusts to respond to 95% of category B calls within 14(urban)/19(rural) minutes
- Maintain a 2-week maximum wait from urgent GP referral to first outpatient appointment for all urgent suspected cancer referrals
- Maintain a maximum 2-week wait standard for Rapid Access Chest Pain Clinics
- A 3-month maximum wait for revascularization by March 2005
- From April 2002, all patients who have operations cancelled for non-clinical reasons to be offered another binding date within 28 days or fund the patient's treatment at the time and hospital of the patient's choice

[a] Reproduced from reference 8. Department of Health © Crown Copyright 2004.

It is incumbent upon medical directors to understand, follow and interpret this process locally. They will wish to ensure that their organizations are not taken by surprise by proposals from the Commission and are prepared to demonstrate how the organization not only gets the basics right but also is making and sustaining progress.

Trust declarations

The Healthcare Commission makes it very clear that, in their declaration on the extent to which they meet core standards, each Trust has to include the views of patients and other partners in the local health economy. Again, medical directors and other senior managers have a vital role to play in

---

TABLE 8.5 Commitments due to be achieved after March 2005[a]

- Improve life and outcomes of adults and children with mental health problems by ensuring that all patients who need them have access to crisis services by 2005, and a comprehensive child and adolescent mental health service by 2006
- Ensure that by the end of 2005, every hospital appointment will be booked for the convenience of the patient, making it easier for patients and their GPs to choose the hospital and consultant that best meets their needs. By December 2005, patients will be able to choose from at least four or five different healthcare providers for planned hospital care, paid for by the NHS
- Ensure a maximum waiting time of 1 month from diagnosis to treatment for all cancers by December 2005
- Achieve a maximum waiting time of 2 months from urgent referral to treatment for all cancers by December 2005
- 800 000 smokers from all groups successfully quitting at the 4-week stage by 2006
- In primary care, update practice-based registers so that patients with CHD and diabetes continue to receive appropriate advice and treatment in line with NSF standards and, by March 2006, ensure practice-based registers and systematic treatment regimes, including appropriate advice on diet, physical activity and smoking, also cover the majority of patients at high risk of CHD, particularly those with hypertension, diabetes and a BMI greater than 30
- A minimum of 80% of people with diabetes to be offered screening for the early detection (and treatment if needed) of diabetic retinopathy by 2006, and 100% by 2007
- Achieve a maximum wait of 3 months for an outpatient appointment by December 2005
- Achieve a maximum wait of 6 months for inpatients by December 2005
- Deliver a 10 percentage-point increase per year in the proportion of people suffering from a heart attack who receive thrombolysis within 60 minutes of calling for professional help
- Delayed transfers of care to reduce to a minimal level by 2006

---

[a] Reproduced from reference 8. Department of Health © Crown Copyright 2004.

communicating what is happening within the Trust to these external stakeholders.

Other statutory bodies

One important new aspect of these ratings is that they will take into account any adverse finding made by other statutory bodies, such as the Health and Safety Executive. Medical directors need to ensure that they are aware of and exercise their statutory responsibilities, particularly with regard to health and safety. For instance, demonstration that their organization has proper procedures in place for training in decontamination and in the maintenance of medical equipment is just one area for which they may be held responsible.

Leadership

In addition, the Healthcare Commission will be conducting a number of *improvement reviews*, which are topic-based. As a part of their improvement, a review of governance, leadership and organizational capacity will be included. Medical directors are responsible for leading not only their medical colleagues but also, with others, associated multidisciplinary teams.

Those who are currently medical directors will have demonstrated their leadership ability – otherwise they would not be in the post. However, they do have to take responsibility for the development of future leaders within the organization – not just doctors, but also other clinicians and managers. This is a vital function within any successful organization.

It follows that, in order to understand what they will require from others and how they might develop future leaders, medical directors must develop their own leadership abilities.

TABLE 8.6 New national targets

Priority I: Improve the health of the population

By 2010, increased life-expectancy at birth in England to 78.6 years for men and to 82.5 years for women.

- **Substantially reduced mortality rates** by 2010 (from the *Our Healthier Nation* baseline, 1995–97):
  - From heart disease and stroke and related diseases by at least 40% in people under 75, with a 40% reduction in the inequalities gap between the fifth of areas with the worst health and deprivation indicators and the population as a whole

TABLE 8.6 *continued*

- – From cancer by at least 20% in people under 75, with a reduction in the inequalities gap of at least 6% between the fifth of areas with the worst health and deprivation indicators and the population as a whole
- – From suicide and undetermined injury by at least 20%
- **Reduced health inequalities** by 10% by 2010 (from a 1997–99 baseline), as measured by infant mortality and life-expectancy at birth
- **Tackle the underlying determinants of ill-health and health inequalities by:**
  - – Reducing adult smoking rates (from 26% in 2002) to 21% or less by 2010, with a reduction in prevalence among routine and manual groups (from 31% in 2002) to 26% or less
  - – Halting the year-on-year rise in obesity among children under 11 by 2010 (from the 2002–04 baseline) in the context of a broader strategy to tackle obesity in the population as a whole (joint target with the Department for Education and Skills and the Department of Culture, Media and Sport)
  - – reducing the under-18 conception rate by 50% by 2010 (from the 1998 baseline), as part of a broader strategy to improve sexual health (joint target with the Department for Education and Skills)

Priority II: Supporting people with long-term conditions

Improve health outcomes for people with long-term conditions by offering a personalized care plan for vulnerable people most at risk; and to reduce emergency bed days by 5% by 2008 (from the expected 2003–04 baseline), through improved care in primary care and community settings for people with long-term conditions

Priority III: Access to services

- Ensure that by 2000 no one waits more than 18 weeks from GP referral to hospital treatment
- Increase the participation of problem drug users in drug treatment programmes by 100% by 2008 (from a 1998 baseline); and increase year-on-year the portion of users successfully sustaining or completing treatment programmes

Priority IV: Patient/user experience

Secure sustained national improvements in NHS patient experience by 2008, ensuring that individuals are fully involved in decisions about their healthcare, including choice of provider, as measured by independently validated surveys. The experiences of black and minority ethnic groups will be specifically monitored as part of these surveys.

Improve the quality of life and independence of vulnerable older people by supporting them to live in their homes where possible by:

- increasing the proportion of older people being supported to live in their own home by 1% annually in 2007 and 2008
- increasing by 2008 the portion of those supported intensively to live at home to 34% of the total of those being supported at home or in residential care

Achieve the year-on-year reductions in MRSA levels, expanding to cover other healthcare-associated infections as data from mandatory surveillance becomes available

[a] Reproduced from reference 8. Department of Health © Crown Copyright 2004.

The NHS Modernisation Agency Leadership Centre provides a Medical Directors Development Framework, which describes the qualities, behaviours, skills and knowledge required for senior medical roles. These are also available for chief executives, for whom they were originally devised, professional executive chairs and directors of nursing.

The various elements of the medical director's role are described. These are:

- *corporate responsibility* – a shared responsibility for strategic direction across the trust and for driving forward the national and local agenda for healthcare development
- *leadership across the trust* – an ability to translate vision into action, taking into account what is possible and the prevailing culture and political climate
- *managing services and information* – the ability to interpret and manage disparate and complex information in making decisions that impact upon the performance of the trust
- *external relationships* – an ability to successfully manage the diverse range of relationships that a trust maintains with the local community, partners and other stakeholders

The Medical Directors Development Framework has three main aims: to support medical directors already in post, to help aspiring medical directors and to help those appointing and working with medical directors. The profile is based around the NHS Leadership Qualities Framework (Department of Health, 2002) and addresses three clusters of competencies – personal qualities, setting direction and service delivery – to categorize the qualities, knowledge and skills that an effective leader should possess.

Medical directors can have a key influence upon the tone and culture of their organizations. Through their own behaviours, they can set a positive tone, particularly with senior medical staff, about the benefits of change.

At the same time, they have to be demonstrably a part of the corporate team. Within this team, the medical director can have a profound and positive effect upon the quality of care given within the Trust that far exceeds their clinical impact upon their own patients.

Through the relationships that they can develop with key external stakeholders, medical directors can also make a positive impact upon care in the local health economy, particularly if they demonstrate a willingness to put their expertise and experience at the disposal of others.

Medical directors have a very specific leadership role in supporting clinical directors in the management of their services. This will be to provide not only a management function but also coaching and mentorship. While they may not provide these latter services personally, it is incumbent upon them to ensure that they are in place.

Putting it into practice

It is relatively easy to establish mechanisms at the top of an organization to respond to the central demands of performance management, which require measurement of money or activity. The real challenge is to improve the standards of care throughout a large organization by influencing many thousands of employees in a systematic fashion. Medical directors, with their executive colleagues, have this to do if NHS Trusts are going to be able to complete in the healthcare markets of the future. The advent of patient choice, if fully exercised, poses just such a challenge.

It is of interest and concern that in a simulation of the impact of 'Patient Choice' commissioned by the Department of Health, acute Trusts made little attempt to drive up the quality of care as a way of attracting more patients to them.[9] The paper goes on to remark that improving the quality of clinical care and the environment in which it is delivered has to be a 'first-order' response for managers and clinicians in the NHS. Their responsiveness to patient needs and preferences was poor in comparison with a much more astute and creative private sector.

For the service improvement to become an established part of the culture of organizations, medical directors must ensure that appropriate structures are put in place to support clinicians at the patient interface. Cohesive support teams addressing risk, clinical effectiveness and quality improvement should be provided for each directorate or department. These teams should be supported by a central resource of experts in the field of risk management, complaints, litigation, health and safety, blood transfusion, etc. Ideally, they should be a single 'front door' that will sort governance issues, from complaints to whistleblowing, into appropriate streams and manage them.

Central collation enables clear prioritization of issues, the development of appropriate corrective actions, and entry into a risk register at an appropriate level in the organization if the problem is not resolved. Items in the risk register can then be systematically addressed through business planning.

Clinical governance meetings

Participation of clinical staff in governance activities must also be promoted for this process to be effective. Medical directors should ensure that every clinical grouping holds regular multidisciplinary 'clinical governance' meetings, which, among other things, consider aspects of patient outcomes, risk, complaints and claims. Each department should have a clinical governance lead (if appropriate a clinical director), and meetings should have a clinical governance facilitator whose job it is to organize an agenda that addresses the issues pertinent to be that specialty.

At these meetings, debate should take place about the quality of care being provided, informed by statistics on complaints, claims, incidents and the like. Clinicians should be provided with information about the outcomes of their clinical practice. Medical directors should ensure that their organization can provide clinicians with suitable data against which they are able to benchmark their practice. A number of commercial organizations will provide such information, notably *Dr Foster*. They also need to make sure that clinicians are aware of their responsibility to produce information about the work that they do.

The healthcare governance department should also provide a horizon scanning service to inform teams about relevant developments in their area. This should enable them to examine critically the care that they provide and to change in order to remain in the forefront of clinical advance.

Other issues

Medical directors have to ensure that all staff know what standards are expected of them. They must therefore assure themselves that an appropriate range of interrelated policies and procedures are available. A list is provided in

TABLE 8.7 Trust policies and procedures

- Risk management strategy
- Risk management policy
- Serious incident policy
- Consent-to-examination policy
- Records management policy
- Blood transfusion policy
- Management of medical devices
- Medicines code
- Do not attempt resuscitation (DNAR) policy
- Health and safety policy
- Control of infection policy
- Complaints and compliments policy
- Security and confidentiality of patient information
- Whistle-blowing policy
- Disciplinary policy
- Appraisal policy
- Training and development policy
- Human resources (HR) policies and procedures
- Data quality strategy
- Patient involvement strategy
- Innovative procedures and treatments policy

Table 8.7, which is not exhaustive but demonstrates the breadth of expertise required of medical directors.

Conclusion

The range of opportunities available to medical directors to stimulate an improvement in healthcare standards is enormous. At the same time, they need to have a wide knowledge of how the health service operates and a clear understanding of how to lead and promote change. The passion and vision must also be there.

Our health service is a complex adaptive system. Small changes can create large (and sometimes unexpected) effects. The system is populated by highly adaptable elements, clinicians, who will continue to produce a new pattern of behaviours in the face of change. Medical directors, with their extensive experience of the system, are extremely well placed to manage change within the care environment. They are also in the best position to influence the behaviours of clinicians, to change their ways to better meet the needs of patients, and to demonstrate values that will lead to improvement of standards.

Healthcare organizations in the UK are preoccupied with financial survival, and given the advent of foundation trusts, payment by results and patient choice. They are becoming overwhelmed with regulation and, to an increasing degree, with litigation. The enormous challenge for medical directors is to make high quality of care the driver and to focus the attention of clinicians and supporting staff on this aim.

Author's note

As this chapter was being written, a large amount of new material was released by the Department of Health and the Healthcare Commission. Every effort has been made to incorporate this material; however, it is highly likely that more relevant information will become available before this book is published.

References

1. Scally G, Donaldson LJ. Looking forward: clinical governance and the drive for quality improvement in the new NHS in England. *BMJ* 1998; **317:** 61–5.
2. *Governance in the New NHS: Controls Assurance Statements 1999/2000: Risk Management and Organisational Controls.* HSC 1999/123. London: Department of Health, 1999.

3. *Assurance – The Board Agenda*. London: Department of Health, 2003.
4. *Compliance Consultation*. London: Monitor, Independent Regulator of NHS Foundation Trusts, November 2004.
5. *National Standards, Local Action*. Health and Social Care Standards and Planning Framework, 2005/06–2007/08. London: Department of Health, 2004.
6. *Improving Health in Wales. A Statement of Health Care Standards – Standards for NHS Care and Treatment in Wales*. November 2004. NHS Wales, 2004.
7. *Better Information, Better Choices, Better Health. Putting Information at the Centre of Health*. London: Department of Health, December 2004.
8. *Assessment for Improvement – Our Approach. A Consultation Document on the Assessment of the Performance of Healthcare Organisations*. London: Healthcare Commission, November 2004.
9. *Balancing choice. A Report on Simulation Based Learning About the Medium Term Impact of 'Patient Choice' on the NHS*. Commissioned by the Department of Health. London: Office for Public Management, April 2004.

Introduction

For the past 20 years or so, medical education has suffered a continuous revolution from which there is apparently no respite.[1]

For very many years, undergraduate education was subject to the occasional experiment, and it is only recently with political pressure and the demand for more medical practitioners that the universities and the General Medical Council (GMC) have come under heavy obligation to increase the number of medical schools, shorten the medical course and expand the selection process by including disadvantaged applicants and graduates not necessarily from scientific disciplines.[2] Increasingly, undergraduate education is being transferred into the community away from the medical schools and universities.[3]

The pressure for change in postgraduate education has been much more immediate as a result of landmark European legislation – firstly on reduction of the total length of specialist training and then devastatingly through a now-immutable programme of reduction of hours of work. Additional pressures have come through New Labour manifestos to shorten waiting lists for diagnosis and treatment, resulting in pressure on educators to concentrate on service provision. The change in ethos in the goals of medical education is nicely summed up in the quotation 'just in time', rather than 'just in case'.[4]

Until the late 1980s, there had been little change in the form of medical education for several hundred years. The process was experiential, with the quality and quantity of education and training being related to the knowledge and charisma of the trainers and resilience and sense of vocation of the trainees. The process could be very long and dependent on patronage.[5] Entry to each level of seniority was governed by examinations of a very traditional form administered first by the universities (qualifying exams) and subsequently by the Royal Colleges. There were no formal curricula, and for each specialty the syllabus was open-ended.

Supporters of the system maintain that it was time-hallowed and fit for its purpose – but most importantly it tested not only actual knowledge and clinical ability but also professional qualities that were rarely itemized or defined but were apparent to any senior consultant examiner across the green baize.

Critics of the system complained at the lack of standardization and an evidence base for goals and outcomes of the process and at the sheer amateurishness in the conduct of the examinations. Of even more importance was the lack of a curriculum and of any linkage of the examination process with an organized training programme.

Such a system was never likely to be capable of withstanding increasingly disrespectful political interference, particularly when the profession had never considered service provision as the highest priority. But other pressures for change appeared in quick succession and from widely different sources.

'Calmanization'

The goal of harmonization of employment in Europe, with mutual acceptability of training programmes, higher examinations and specialist qualifications, was extended to medicine. In the UK, until the early 1990s, it was not exceptional for the duration of postgraduate training leading to a consultant appointment to be 15 years or more. Elsewhere in Europe, specialist training might be no more than 6 years.

Calman was arguably the first Chief Medical Officer to consider medical training as a major focus for change, although even this was limited to hospital specialist training. In a decade, the old system was replaced as comprehensively as state secondary education had been 20 years before.[6]

While the principal changes were directed towards specialist training, several specialties took the opportunity of reorganizing and more closely defining basic training at SHO level. For example, the Colleges of Surgeons were certainly proactive in defining two-year rotations of six-monthly posts appropriate for basic surgical training and subject to regular inspection by the Colleges but with ultimate responsibility to the Specialist Training Authority (STA). The old two-part FRCS examination evolved into the MRCS with a well-defined syllabus, comprehensive cover of the basic sciences and the fundamental elements of all the surgical specialties, with mandatory courses teaching basic surgical skills, advanced trauma and life support and care of the critically sick patient. A common specialist grade, the SpR, replaced the old grading of registrar and senior registrar. By and large, specialist training was concluded after five or six years, with accreditation and entry onto the specialist register with the right to apply for consultant posts and to practise independently. The hallmark of SpR training was the RITA process (record of in-training assessment) by which the ability of the trainee was signed off by the training committee or alternatively referred for remedial training based on the opinions of the trainer in each six-month training slot.

In the ten years or so of the existence of 'Calman', there have been refinements. It is recognized that ideally at the beginning of every post, an educational contract should be negotiated between trainer and trainee and a formal appraisal initiated through formative and summative assessments with regular mutual feedback. An attempt has been made to standardize training methods through the introduction of 'Training the Trainer' courses and to refine the syllabus by developing a generic curriculum for higher postgraduate clinical training.[7]

There has been growing recognition that some practical skills need to be taught.[8,9]

From the outset, the surgical specialties developed specialist exit examinations termed FRCS, with a suffix describing the specialty. Ultimately, success at the examination became a mandatory element of accreditation.

Criticism of Calman – pressures to change

Calman training has been criticised within the profession for several reasons:[10]

- In the view of some, particularly in the surgical disciplines, limitation of higher surgical training to a maximum of 6 years is insufficient to allow the young consultant to function safely independently. The situation is now exacerbated by the impositions of the European Working Time Directive (EWTD). The new consultant may require a period of mentoring after appointment and therefore is an old-style senior registrar in all but name.
- The process of signing off each six-month attachment is imperfect and cannot necessarily be left to the Medical Royal Colleges, who are responsible for arranging the membership examinations. Neither can quality of the end-result be assured by success in the Intercollegiate Specialty Examination. While there is not necessarily a causal relationship, there are several examples of young consultants suspended by their Trusts on account of poor clinical performance or, more problematically, defects in communication and attitude that should have been detected during training. 'Calman' was introduced as a package deal with no attempt to pilot the more problematic elements. The RITA questionnaire, appraisal and assessment,

particularly of technical skills, received little detailed attention. Also, recognition that not all clinicians have the time, inclination or ability to teach, assess and provide constructive feedback has come surprisingly late in the day. It has not been exceptional for SHOs to pass through an ill-coordinated collection of six-month posts that prepare them poorly for the membership examinations and thereafter the higher surgical training in specialist registrar posts.

- Manpower predictions were always notoriously inaccurate. Bottlenecks always seem to have occurred at the SHO/registrar interface, and now, in the desirable specialties, it is not exceptional for there to be fifty SHO applications received for one SpR post. At the other end of the production line in the same desirable specialty, there may be insufficient accredited trainees to fill the consultant posts. The Chief Medical Officer showed his displeasure at the poor quality of SHO teaching and the need for change.[11]

The Government and Civil Service have also grown restive at the inability of the universities, Royal Colleges, Deaneries and GMC to deliver compliant and skilful practitioners in sufficient numbers to satisfy political imperatives. A greater revolution still than Calman, 'Modernising Medical Careers' is planned to redress the balance.

Controls and validation

The revolution in medical practice has also embodied increasing awareness that patients may suffer positive harm at the hands of their medical practitioners. No doubt, when the history of the NHS is written, the Bristol Paediatric Cardiac Surgery debacle culminating in the Kennedy Report will, together with a number of other notorious cases, appear to be the impetus for an explosion of quality control, incident reporting and the study of risk and the establishment by government of a variety of Quangos. In fact, the public recognition of fallibility within the medical profession as a basis for medico-legal action has been an increasing fact of life over the past two decades. After years of relative inactivity, the GMC has been obliged to react with a series of edicts defining the ethical and professional basis for practice (e.g. 'Tomorrow's Doctors') and reinterpreted by the Royal Colleges to define the specialist aspects of professionalism. The obligation to submit results of treatment to a process of audit both individually and through various national initiatives (e.g. CEPOD) was established before Bristol, but it must be admitted that the pace has quickened since then.

The publication of data relating to quality of performance by clinicians individually and corporately within the NHS system is now regularly undertaken, and inevitably the development of league tables is a natural consequence. Unfortunately, there is an astonishing lack of awareness of simple statistics and of the influence of varying case mix in practice, so that the analysis may be crude and misleading. Nevertheless, the principle is laudable, and the validity can only improve with public education. There is an urgent need for clinicians to collect and classify data on diagnosis, treatment and outcome of care, and this is slowly being addressed.

There seems little doubt that the work of the future doctor will be governed by attention to guidelines, protocols, benchmarks and an evidence base whose validity has been formally classified.[12] The future doctor will regard the frank discussion of a patient's disease, efficacy of treatment, and analysis of risks and benefits as second nature. Both doctor and patient will have free access to the Internet, and much of the clinician's responsibility will devolve on interpretation of the evidence so that consent will be genuinely informed.

The modern doctor will be much more prepared to accept the moderating influence of the team and the system on clinical practice than his or her multiskilled predecessor. The Calman trainee and the product of even shorter programmes in the future will not wish to work independently, but will submit to corporate opinion formulated by a multidisciplinary team. Similarly, he or she would understand that malfunction of a system rather than an individual is responsible for an adverse incident.

The European Working Time Directive[13,14]

Intuitively, long hours of work and chronic fatigue will lead to poor performance. There is also a body of evidence demonstrating a direct relationship between sleep deprivation and a whole range of physiological consequences and performance indicators.[15,16] These issues were recognized early on, and the New Deal emerged in 1991 as a recommendation that the maximum number of hours worked, including prospective holiday cover, should be 72 hours per week but average out to no more than 56 hours.

For the traditionalist, a reduction of hours worked in the week together with limitation of the total period of specialist training will inevitably lead to a lack of awareness of the importance of continuity of care and of experience in managing the whole range of emergencies and complications that will of course only occur sporadically. In the UK, such a wealth of experience could only be picked up by chance meandering through up to 15 years of specialist instruction. Elsewhere, superior training could be acquired in a much more concentrated form, as perfected in the USA from a six-year residency in a university teaching hospital with training programmes directed by faculty, staff and the 'attendings', with the opportunity to practise what had been learnt in the local Veterans Administration hospital.

The European Working Time Directive regulations were introduced in October 1998. Initially, various 'derogations' were accepted such that the restrictions need not apply to doctors in training. However, in August 2004, a limit of 58 hours per week (decreasing to 56 hours by August 2007 and 48 hours by 2009) were set by legislation in the European Parliament, with appropriate sanctions for non-compliance. In some countries, this had been anticipated and solutions had been evolved in good time. In the UK, an attitude of something between weary acceptance and blind panic has been pervasive. Undoubtedly, introduction of the Directive represents a large component of the revolution in training for future doctors and specialists, but the tendency has been for consultants and junior staff to unite in looking for faults rather than solutions and sharing the same delusion of a 'folie à deux'. A commonly quoted calculation has shown that pre-Calman specialists would have undergone approximately 22 000 hours of training, the Calman trainee 15 000 hours and those training after 2004, 6000 hours. On the other hand, a minority recognize that the change can be used as an opportunity for the public's benefit in altering the delivery of service through reconfiguration of specialties within the health service and dismantling of the tiers of junior staffing and the hierarchy of care.

What is work? The consequences of the full shift on training

The definition of 'What is Work' has recently come under scrutiny with a *cause célèbre* in Spain. As a result, the European Directive has determined that working is not just when the worker is working but also when he or she is at the disposal of the employer. In other words, rest on call at home is 'work' even if it is invariably uninterrupted. It was therefore decided that in every 24-hour period, the worker should have at least 11 hours away from the workplace. The consequence for medical training has been that it is rarely possible to provide on-call cover, and a full shift system is inevitably leading to fewer training opportunities – particularly in specialties where all of the elective work and formal education are arranged during daylight hours.[17]

In surgery, it has been recognized that many of the emergencies that were customarily operated on an all-night emergency list could be left until the following day. One of the recommendations of CEPOD was the establishment of the daytime emergency theatre staffed by a surgical team with no responsibilities for elective work. This experience will clearly no longer be available for the trainee on the nightshift.

The disadvantage of the full shift is that the individual may, in the short term (over the course of a week or so), work much longer hours when, for example, working a week of nights with all the well-rehearsed consequences of disrupted diurnal rhythm.[18,19] Another disadvantage is that most rotas divide the weekends and daytime working into early and late shifts, with a reduction in the number of full weekends off duty. This again can affect incumbents' social life. A week of nights is followed by a week off duty, again restricting learning and training opportunities.

At present, virtually all of the PRHO and SHO rotations have been altered to a full shift, while SpRs have been allowed to remain on an on-call rota. However, the time spent on duty will then be heavily influenced by how busy the nights are. It has been estimated that time at work could be reduced by as much as 30%. Ultimately, with the reduction to 48 hours, a full shift is inevitable at all levels, possibly including consultants in busy specialties.

It may be concluded that the simple well-intentioned reduction of working hours has done little to ameliorate the perennial problem for doctors of stress at work.[20,21]

Staffing of a hospital through the full 24-hour period may require more than the total number of official trainees available. The number can be made up with so-called 'clinical fellows', some of whom will be mainly occupied in research posts. Alternatively, SAS doctors (staff grades and associated specialists) can be employed, although this is usually unsatisfactory as it is professionally unrewarding for the incumbent and an expensive solution to night cover for the Trust. Other possibilities include cross-cover with other specialties. This is generally regarded as unacceptable for higher-level as opposed to basic-level trainees. On the other hand, there may be an advantage for more junior doctors to experience exposure and training in a variety of acute specialties.

The hospital at night

With the development of on-call daytime emergency teams, it is recognized in surgery, and to a lesser extent in other acute specialties, that there are fewer emergency admissions during the night and that only a small proportion of these require immediate surgical treatment. It is also recognized that the general level of activity in the hospital at 5 AM is one-quarter of that at 4 PM, but staffing levels still do not necessarily reflect this. Accordingly, this has led to the development of the 'Hospital at Night' model by the Joint Consultants Committee with representation by the Academy of Royal Colleges and the British Medical Association (BMA).[22] The plan is to have one or more multidisciplinary teams providing a full range of skills and urgent care beyond the responsibility of the Accident and Emergency Department.[23] Further research has indicated that medical problems arising in patients admitted under all specialties represent the majority of the night-time workload, but in general there are few calls for middle-grade staff in surgery or orthopaedics. Reduction in night-time operating has obvious implications for anaesthetic services. The possibility of withdrawing anaesthetists from the 'crash' team subject to sufficient non-anaesthetic staff being able to provide airway management skills remains.

The initiative will consider the use of doctors from other specialties who have been trained to have the appropriate competencies and of nurse practitioners and support staff to undertake particular tasks such as triage, airway management, infection control, prescribing within defined protocols, venepuncture and cannulation, and urethral catheterization. Increasingly, these tasks will be undertaken by operating department assistants and the outreach nursing team.

It is clear from the pilot studies that a review of night-time working in any hospital can offer considerable benefits in hospital management and patient care. It is obviously important that data are collected locally to determine the clinical workload at night and an agreement reached on the competencies required to manage that night-time workload. The leadership of the night team will need to be determined, but effective handover and transfer of cases, together with redefinition or emphasis of bleep policies, are all likely to have a knock-on benefit during daytime hours. This initiative will have some impact on training, as arguably there will be less opportunity for the junior surgeon or physician to acquire skills 'creamed off' by the emergency night team.

Modernizing medical careers (MMC) (middle-grade medical crisis!)[24]

The present Government above all resolved to reduce waiting lists for diagnosis and treatment. The obvious solution was a rapid increase in the number of specialists trained to deal with the elective conditions, mainly within the surgical specialties. The Department of Health and the Treasury were prepared to increase spending on the NHS to £100 billion (9% of the Gross Domestic Product by 2007), but were frustrated by the gross deficit in availability of trained staff. In their scrutiny of the existing system of training and hospital staffing, they strangely found common ground with much of the medical profession (Table 9.1).

TABLE 9.1 Deficiencies of existing training and regulation prior to MMC

- Chronic inadequacy of manpower calculations
- Inappropriate content and length of undergraduate and postgraduate medical education for ultimate service
- Obduracy of the Royal Colleges and their plethora of training and assessment committees in adjusting education to service needs or in tolerating any external control of training
- Failure of organization, leading in particular to poor quality of basic training in medicine and surgery and in selection of posts often not 'fit for purpose'
- Proliferation of inspection committees reporting to the Royal Colleges and Deaneries, with little coordination of effort or standardization of the process and poor quality of reporting
- Inadequate management of risk, incident reporting and medical governance. Failure of a system of control and a review of medical performance within the medical profession (i.e. the GMC)

The curriculum[25]

The complete revision of medical training began with a paper by the Chief Medical Officer outlining deficiencies of the SHO training grade.[11] It has rapidly evolved to provide a common pathway that can be adapted to the needs of medical specialties.[26]

The plan was influenced by educational medical theorists and by the need to minimize medical training so that it was fit for purpose (to provide service needs). A general outline of the training plan is shown in Figure 9.1. It begins with two foundation years, with F1, the equivalent to the PRHO year, leading to full registration by proving to the GMC competency to practise. However, F1 and F2 should be seen as a continuum providing 2–4 months' exposure to a wide range of specialties, some of which would not have been included in previous schemes at such an early stage (e.g. anaesthetics, microbiology, general practice and ITU). Generic, clinical, personal and professional skills formalized in a curriculum will be tested through a series of 'competencies' and other assessments. Their acquisition will allow passage through to F3. This year could mark the beginning of 'run-through' training for high-fliers and trainees who are certain of their choice of specialty, aptitude and abilities or as a time for review and movement between posts of more conventional SHO form. All of the subsequent years up to F7 will be structured, with an extension of the curriculum and a specific syllabus for basic and specialist training. Figure 9.2 shows how the template can be applied to surgical training. The position of formal examinations is likely to be at the end of year 4, although seamless training within any particular specialty could entail a

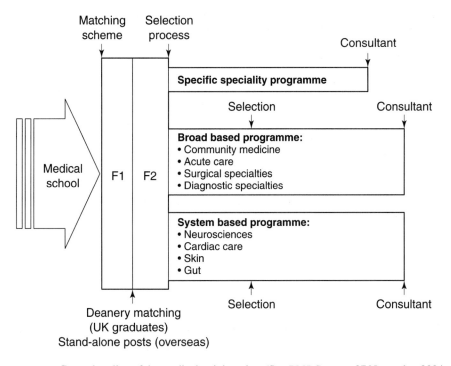

FIGURE 9.1 General outline of the medical training plan. (See *BMJ Careers*, 27 November 2004, p. 217)

different format (e.g. urology[27]). Currently F1 is being piloted with a general introduction in August 2005. There is as yet some uncertainty among final-year medical students as to the content of their F2 posts.

The core curriculum for the foundation years emphasizes the diagnosis and management of the acutely ill patient with clinical governance, patient safety, infection control, teamwork and the patient's personal experience as the five linchpins for securing high-quality clinical care. A framework of the curriculum defined for surgical training by the JCHST emphasizes standards to be established and assessed at every stage in clinical judgement, technical and operative skills, specialty-based knowledge and generic professional skills. The foundation training aims to establish 'a new generation of doctors who early in their careers are characterized by the behaviours, attitudes and values required for excellent healthcare interactions with patients, their carers and their families.' Such noble aims expressed in this credo might be said to state the obvious and should always have been the foundation of medical training and even firmly established at an undergraduate level.

The curriculum document also emphasizes ward-based learning, supervised consultations in outpatient clinics and, where relevant, practical instruction in

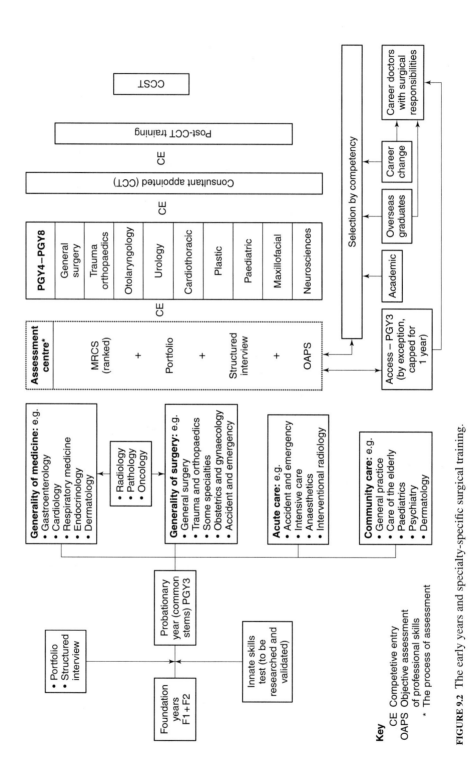

Key
CE   Competetive entry
OAPS   Objective assessment
         of professional skills
*   The process of assessment

FIGURE 9.2 The early years and specialty-specific surgical training.

the operating theatre. What is new is the obligation to record all such learning experiences and feedback in a portfolio that might subsequently be used for validation. In addition, the core competencies relating to management of the acutely ill patient[28] will have explicit incremental standards based on the management of a variety of common clinical presentations. Increasingly, simulated clinical environments will be used. The principles of evidence-based medicine will be formally taught to direct selection of treatment according to formulated guidelines.[12] In addition four assessment tools will be used at various times during each placement to a total of approximately four and a half hours. Finally, generic qualities and skills listed by the GMC in the 'New Doctor', 'Good Medical Practice' and 'Good Surgical Practice'[29] will be continually re-emphasized through F1, F2 and beyond.

While the publication of plans for F1 and F2 have been welcomed optimistically, there is on the contrary much disquiet that the system may not deliver a competent specialist eight years after qualification (Table 9.2). This

TABLE 9.2 The new training plan in MMC – for and against

Pro

- Early exposure to a variety of specialties (F2)
- Structured training with emphasis on acquisition of skills, attitudes and communication
- Formal competency testing and other regular assessments in a portfolio
- Formal teaching of the principles of risk assessment and incident reporting
- Appraisal and feedback
- Educational contracts
- One-to-one consultant/trainer teaching in the outpatient clinic and operating theatre facilitated by 'hot weeks' on call
- Evidence-based treatment
- CEPOD

Con

- Shortening of training period
- EWTD
- Increase in numbers of personnel
- Waiting list initiatives
- Independent treatment centres
- Day surgery undertaken by consultants
- Absence of parallel operating lists
- Shift working/lack of continuity of care and training
- Consultant-led service
- Surgical nurse assistants
- High public expectation – threat of retribution – zero tolerance of complications
- Inflexible guidelines
- Subspecialization

feeling of insecurity is particularly prevalent in general surgery, where such an individual has already been termed under MMC proposals as an 'emergency safe surgeon'.[30] Increasing subspecialization within the generic confines of 'general surgery' would undoubtedly mean that specialists undergoing fast-track training to year 8 in breast, vascular and upper gastrointestinal surgery would not be available for cross-specialty cover. Supporters of MMC have strongly denied that the trainees under the new system would be less experienced at the time of accreditation with the CBST. They have suggested that the new system of competency-based training would mean that time would not be wasted on skills that were not necessary for their chosen specialty.

Seamless training in urology – a controversial experiment

Some of the doubts and conundrums of MMC in the light of changing practice have been specifically addressed by urologists.[27] Due recognition has been given to 'medicalization' of what was hitherto a surgical specialty into a subspecialization such that fewer more extensive operative procedures need to be concentrated on small teams of urological surgeons. And yet, a greater number of 'specialists' overall is required to investigate increasing numbers of patients with symptoms that might arise in the genitourinary tract but for whom medication is the first appropriate treatment and of steeply rising numbers of patients presenting with symptoms that might indicate the presence of genitourinary malignancy. In such patients, there are very many false positives, and even if the diagnosis is secured, a surgical treatment may not necessarily be appropriate.

There has been a great deal of discussion as to whether non-surgical urologists should undergo primarily surgical training or should take up a newly devised training plan beginning two or three years after F2. Currently, the provisional plan is that such individuals, who will represent the majority of trainees, will become certified as specialists in urology and will have achieved competence in advanced ultrasound imaging, prostatic biopsy and urodynamic assessment, and in inguino-scrotal surgery and minor endoscopy, including the diagnosis of bladder tumours and transurethral resection of small prostates.

Urologists who wish to become urological surgeons will, after acquisition of the CBST, compete for three-year training fellowships in one of the four urological subspecialties. These include advanced endourology, including the majority of urinary stone management, urological oncology, female and reconstructive urology, and andrology. Arguably, renal transplantation –

currently a general surgical subspecialty that is experiencing great difficulty in attracting trainees – should once again become a urological surgical subspecialty with its own three-year higher surgical training programme attracting an input from either general surgical or urological core specialists.

The introduction of seamless training is also being considered in other specialties in much the same way as postgraduate training is organized in the USA. It can obviously be tailored to provide a very efficient focused form of training at the expense of breadth and flexibility.[31]

PMETB

The Postgraduate Medical Education and Training Board was set up under the General and Specialist Medical Practice Order 2003.[32] There seems little question that it was established by the Government to oversee medical education, training and assessment within the context of MMC and ultimately to absorb the roles (and many would say the raison d'etre) of the Medical Royal Colleges. Of course, this process may take many years, and the PMETB may never have more than a nominal supervisory function when the Colleges have developed such considerable expertise in training and assessment. Indeed, their willingness to cooperate in modernization by the development of curricula and specialist training and with innovations in assessment at F2 and with higher postgraduate training examinations brings the validity of a new organization into question.

Presently, both the Chief Executive and Chairman of the PMETB have been replaced less than two years after its establishment. It would seem that its first responsibility is to supervise the transfer of appropriately qualified non-career-grade doctors to specialist status under so-called Article 14. There will be an urgent requirement for a plan to be implemented for the Government to keep its promise in appointing new specialists. Otherwise, modest increases can only arise in national training numbers for current SpRs trained conventionally and the few who will pass into the new training system under transitional arrangements. The next wave will not come until the first block of new-system trainees specialize in 2013.

Initiative lists and independent treatment centres

Other possible solutions to increasing the throughput of work and particularly the management of surgical referrals is through the so-called initiative list of patients from the body of long waiters on the NHS waiting list to take up spare capacity in the private sector. This perplexing doctrinal volte-face by the Government has been welcomed by NHS consultants as an extra source of income without the overheads of maintaining a private practice.

The alternative to improve production is the Independent Sector Treatment Centre (ISTC). In 2003, the Government announced successful bids for contracts worth over £2 billion to provide elective surgery for NHS patients performed in the ISTCs with the provision of approximately 120 000 additional procedures by 2005. Until now, these centres have been staffed to perform mainly joint replacement and cataract surgery by teams from Europe and South Africa. It remains to be seen whether this extraordinary innovation can be sustained, but if so then issues surrounding quality control, governance and continuity of care will need to be considered. At present, neither the patients on initiative lists nor those admitted to the ISTCs are available as a teaching resource. This will need to be urgently resolved, as such patients are likely to have less comorbidity and to require more straightforward procedures than those kept on the waiting list for surgery in NHS hospitals. They are therefore optimal patients for supervised training.

Do physician/nursing assistants pose a threat to medical trainees?

Rather gratuitously, it is said that the defining features of a surgeon as opposed to the pure technician are the qualities of knowledge, judgement and accountability.[33] There seems little question that nurses, operating department assistants and others with medical training considerably shorter and more limited than their surgeon and physician counterparts, can be trained to perform efficiently an increasing range of surgical procedures. Using well-established protocols and guidelines, there seems to be no reason why such individuals should not function independently for case selection, treatment evaluation and audit. The principle of others undertaking medical tasks of increasing complexity is now well established in many countries, including the USA.[34] In the UK, the specialist nurse practitioner is familiar in medical and surgical investigation. For some time in cardiac surgery, nurse assistants have been responsible for removing vein grafts, opening and closing the chest, and even establishing the patient on bypass. They are also performing minor orthopaedic procedures most efficiently. It is often said that the day-case unit is an ideal environment for training young surgeons, particularly at an early stage in their career. Many of these minor procedures could also be suitable for nurse practitioners.

In the future, the trainee surgeon should take nothing for granted and must certainly regard non-medically qualified practitioners as a challenge – at least in the acquisition of work experience.

Postscript – educating the doctors of the future

This question has been posed by the GMC to professionals and the public in a project to determine how sociological and technical developments might alter public expectation of the function of the medical practitioner and direct radical changes in training.[35] It is likely that great strides in imaging will continue, allowing the process of diagnosis to become a technical exercise. In consequence, the importance of clinical skills will diminish. Conventional surgical treatment will continue to be eroded by the skills of the interventional radiologist and the laparoscopic surgical expert guided by robotics. An increasingly important element of surgical training will be assessment of aptitude to perform these highly specialized procedures, although the use of sophisticated simulators[36] and virtual reality models will facilitate training and assessment.[37] And yet, with such technological developments, it is likely that the time for interaction between the specialist and patient will be strictly limited. In these circumstances, the role of the general practitioner with his, or increasingly her, well-developed communication skills may assume greater importance as the conductor of the great orchestra.

References

1. Chantler C. The second greatest benefit to mankind. *Lancet* 2002; **360:** 1830–77.
2. Education Committee of the General Medical Council. *Tomorrow's Doctors*. London: General Medical Council, 2002.
3. Worley P, Esterman A, Prideaux D. Cohort study of examination performance of undergraduate medical students learning in a community setting. *BMJ* 2004; **328:** 207–9.
4. Gallen D, Peile E. A firm foundation for senior house officers. *BMJ* 2004; **328:** 1390–1.
5. Goodwin DP. A 'Calman' trainee retires in a professional lifetime of changes in surgical training and practice. *Ann R Coll Surg Engl* 2001; **83:** 355–7
6. Calman KC. *A Guide to Specialist Registrar Training*. London: NHS Executive, Department of Health, 1996.
7. *The New Doctor. Recommendations for a General Clinical Training*. London: General Medical Council, 1997: s 109.
8. Treasure T. Surgeons' knots: old skills, new training. *Lancet* 2002; **359:** 642.
9. Sarker SK. Courses, cadavers and counsellors: reducing errors in the operating theatre. *BMJ Careers* 4 October 2003.
10. Spitz L, Kiely EM, Piero A *et al.* Decline in surgical training. *Lancet* 2002; **359:** 83.

11. Donaldson I. *Unfinished Business. Proposals for the Senior House Officer Grade.* NHS Consultation Paper. London: Department of Health, August 2002.
12. Del Mar C, Glaszion P, Mayer D. Teaching evidence based medicine. *BMJ* 2004; **329:** 989–90.
13. Career Focus. *BMJ Careers* 31 August 2002: 65–72.
14. Eaton L. The European Working Time Directive, the final countdown. *BMJ Careers* 5 June 2004: 229.
15. Tucker P, Folkard S, MacDonald I. Rest breaks and accident risk. *Lancet* 2003; **361:** 680.
16. Hill J. Conduct and compassion – sleep deprivation. *Lancet* 2004; **363:** 996.
17. Davies RJ. Shift work and surgical training. *Ann R Coll Surg Engl* 2004; **86**(Suppl): 85.
18. Costa G. Shift work and occupational medicine – an overview. *Occup Med* 2003; **53:** 83–8.
19. Hobson J. Shift work and doctors' health. *BMJ Careers* 9 October 2004: 149–50.
20. Firth-Cozens J. Doctors, their wellbeing and their stress. *BMJ* 2003; **326:** 670–1.
21. Editorial. *Ann Surg* 2002; **236:** 699–702.
22. *Hospital at Night.* London: Department of Health, 2004.
23. Sykes TCF, Fox AD. Changing times: Doctors at night. *Ann R Coll Surg Engl* 2005; **86:** 314–15.
24. *Modernising Medical Careers. The Response of the Four UK Health Ministers to the Consultation of Unfinished Business.* London: Department of Health, February 2003.
25. *Curriculum for the Foundation Years in Postgraduate Education and Training – a Paper for Consultation.* Academy of Medical Royal Colleges, October 2004.
26. *The Next Steps – the Future Shape of Foundation Specialists' and General Practice Training Programmes.* London: Department of Health, 2004.
27. Mundy AR. Redesigning urological training and the consultant urologist. *Ann R Coll Surg Engl* 2003; **85:** 314–17.
28. Gonizi A. A competence based assessment in the professions in Australia. *Assess Educ* 1994; **1:** 27–44.
29. *Good Medical Practice.* London: General Medical Council, 2001.
30. Watkin DFL, Layer GT. Service and not training for the general surgical SpR on call. *Ann R Coll Surg Engl* 2003; **85:** 310–13.
31. Sher L, Flood L, Plusa S, Waugh L. Developing a seamless training programme for a single deanery. *Bull R Coll Surg Engl* 2004; **86:** 268–70.
32. MacDonald R. The Postgraduate Medical Education and Training Board (PMETB): the view from the top. *BMJ Career Focus* 2004; **328:** 103–5.
33. Nashef SAM. What makes a surgeon? *Ann R Coll Surg Engl* 1999; **81**(Suppl): 44–45.
34. Mettman DE, Cawley JF, Fenn WH. Physician assistants in the United States. *BMJ* 2002; **325:** 485–7.
35. Bulstrode C. What does the future hold? *GMC News* August 2004; **25:** 4–5.
36. Torkington J, Smith SGT, Rees BI, Darzi A. The role of simulation in surgical training. *Ann R Coll Surg Engl* 2000; **82:** 88–94.
37. Gallagher AG, Cotes CU. Virtual reality training for the operating room and cardiac catheterisation laboratory. *Lancet* 2004; **364:** 1538–40.

10 Publishing individual surgical mortality rates

Tom Treasure and Steve Gallivan

This chapter synthesizes the views of a cardiothoracic surgeon (TT) and a non-clinician (SG) who is an expert in operations research, a branch of mathematics concerned with the analysis of complex systems with the aim of improving them. The clinical examples will be biased towards heart and lung surgery because that is where the first author's clinical experience lies. We have tried to make sure that the questions that we raise can be readily translated to all surgery, but it is not unreasonable that we look at it from the heart surgeons' point of view because it is they who are currently under the hammer. We will take the title apart and look first at the question of publishing – which we will consider as meaning in the public domain and accessible to all. We will then consider whether it is better to name or not name the individual surgeon. Finally, we will challenge the implicit belief that mortality rates for operations are useful as isolated information.

Some background: the 'B' word

We have been involved as 'experts' for various enquiries into surgical performance. When we started collecting our thoughts for this chapter, we agreed between ourselves that we would strive to avoid bringing out specific difficult and painful issues. In particular, we started out with the intention of not mentioning Bristol. This has proved impossible. We would fail in the task set for us by the editors if we did not confront the challenges in the Bristol Inquiry and the consequent obligations put upon surgeons by the then Secretary of State, Mr Alan Milburn. At various points, we will use the 'B' word. The legacy of Bristol is inescapable.

Data in the public domain

Openness is not only inevitable – it is right

The emphasis in the Bristol Inquiry was to serve the best interests of patients, and it will be the test that we will use as we consider the various issues throughout our chapter. Will named surgeons' mortality figures in the public domain benefit patients? There is a lot in that question, so let us leave naming and mortality aside and ask one question at a time. To simplify the question and put it another way, what justification could there be for concealment? For a detailed and considered analysis of the general proposition, read Atul Gawande in *The New Yorker*.[1] Gawande describes the experience of the family of a child – he calls her Annie – with cystic fibrosis. The gene for cystic fibrosis is recessive and so the disease crops up unexpectedly if both parents are carriers. Carriers (and there are many because it has a frequency of 1:25) are completely well. For those with cystic fibrosis, secretions throughout the body are thickened. The lethal effects are in the lungs, which are prone to repeated infection. In addition, thick secretions block the pancreatic ducts and the children suffer progressively severe malabsorption and failure to thrive. Not so long ago, most died in childhood, but in 1986–87 the median survival was 25 years in the UK and 30 years in Canada and the USA.[2] The estimate given to Annie's family in 1990s America was that she might see 40. As far as they could judge, and within their sphere of understanding, the hospital was taking the greatest imaginable care of Annie. They assumed that its results were as good as any. What they had to discover for themselves was that their hospital was well below average. It turned out that patients in the care of Annie's hospital had measurements of lung function – a critical indicator of well-being and prognosis – in the lowest quartile compared with similar-aged patients in other hospitals. Gawande assesses the implications of that revelation; it seems inescapable that the data should be freely available. But the process of lifetime management of cystic fibrosis has many events, many decisions and involves many therapists. This is in marked contrast to surgery, where the main issues may be seen as a single event and its outcome. In the arterial switch operation (one of the operations under particular scrutiny in Bristol), the operation can result in life or death. It is an irrevocable intervention at a point in time and the surgeon is centre stage in the operating theatre. It is easier to count and to allocate blame, but does that make it appropriate to do so? For high-risk surgery, death is an obvious outcome to start with, but it is not a good way to judge clinical benefit, and may not be the best way to monitor performance. We will return to that. We will also consider whether naming the surgeon alone out of all the team providing care is a positive contribution. Setting those issues aside for now, openness about surgical outcomes seems to have an inescapable logic. Gawande concludes that openness is unavoidable in something as multifaceted as the care of cystic fibrosis, and it would now be impossible to justify secrecy about surgical mortality. But while openness is to be applauded, it is not that simple. Care has to be taken about what data are reported and how they are presented and interpreted.

Counting and accountability

Annual reports of the results of surgery were provided over 100 years ago, for example by St Thomas' Hospital, which published figures for those who were discharged cured, relieved, unrelieved or who died[3] (Figure 10.1). There was a plea from Bristol in 1908 for the uniform reporting of surgical results.[4] Counting and accountability are an integral part of the history of cardiac surgery, which is largely contained in the second half of the 20th century. There were many instances where surgery advanced by trial and error – and error in this instance means high death rates. When a new operation is tried, or an emerging technology is being developed, there may well be casualties, and when the organ being operated upon is the heart, technical failure translates into deaths. When those deaths are of children, emotions run high. Over the years, the profession and the informed public have understood the difficulties and applauded 'the courage to fail'. In some instances, a procedure is abandoned after a series of failures. In some, there has been a moratorium and the problem is returned to later.[5] Ten or so operations for mitral stenosis were performed in the 1920s,[6] with only two survivors;* surgeons returned to the problem in the 1940s and it became established.[7] The flurry of heart transplants all around the world in the late 1960s was halted until the late 1970s.[5] There was no secret about the identity of any of the surgeons involved, which were in the public arena. Where failure has been openly declared and analysed, it has brought only credit to those concerned.[8] In summary, within surgery, there has been a culture of critical analysis to find the evidence on which to base refinements.[9]

'A failure to act on concerns about services'

So why did this not happen in Bristol? Kennedy found that 'Bristol was awash with data', but the evidence suggested that there were conscious and deliberate

---

* This paper is interestingly entitled 'Present status of surgical procedures in chronic valvular disease of the heart; final report of all surgical cases' and marks the start of the moratorium.

SURGICAL REPORT.

1900.

———

By EDRED M. CORNER, B.Sc.Lond., M.A., M.B., B.C.Cantab.,
F.R.C.S.Eng.,

SURGICAL REGISTRAR.

————

General Surgical Statement.

Number of surgical beds   262

„   of surgical patients in hospital, January 1st 1900 { Males   132
{ Females   76

Total 208

„   „   „   „   December 31st, 1900 { Males   148
{ Females   93

Total 241

„   „   „   treated to a termination in 1900   3317

	Total.		Males.		Females.
Discharged cured	2315	...	1350	...	965
„ relieved . . .	624	...	399	...	225
„ unrelieved . . .	158	...	97	...	61
Died	220	...	140	...	80
Totals	3317		1986		1331

Average number of days in hospital – 21.72.
Death rate = 5.3 per cent.

FIGURE 10.1 Presentation of annual surgical outcomes from 1900[3]

moves to prevent the dissemination of information. From 1992, Dr Philip Hammond was contributing to *Private Eye*.[10] Hammond's view was that while *Private Eye* was publishing alarming stories, members of the surgical and management staff were in denial. His statement to the inquiry repeatedly indicates a lack of openness. It is our impression that the hospital's ethos revealed by the inquiry paved the way to the subsequent commitment to publish cardiac surgery mortality figures. This requirement was reported to Parliament by Mr Milburn on 18 July 2001 in his statement on the Bristol Royal Infirmary Report:[11]

'...the report identifies a failure to act on concerns about services, not through a lack of data, because Bristol was awash with data. There was however, no single point where data were brought together for analysis, evaluation, dissemination, and, most important, follow-up action. For data on surgical outcomes to be published, of course, they need to be robust, rigorous and risk-adjusted. That will inevitably take time. The report does, however, recommend publication to give both NHS staff and the public accurate information. It recommends the establishment of a new independent office for information on health care performance within the Commission for Health Improvement to co-ordinate the collection and publication of data. We will action those two recommendations. In so doing, we will ensure that the new office works in tandem with the medical organisations that have been pioneering improvements on data collection about clinical outcomes.'

It is interesting to note that Mr Milburn's statement to the House of Commons[11] did not include the requirement for named surgeon data. That was made behind the scenes (B Keogh, Personal communication, 1 March 2005: 'Milburn never publicly stated that we needed named surgeon data. This came from private conversations between him, the CMO and the PM's Senior Policy Advisor at No. 10'). However, it is Bristol that was the starting point, and preventing 'another Bristol' is the continued justification for the demand to see named surgeon data published. Again we cannot avoid the 'B' word, for this is considered to be 'the legacy of Bristol'.[12] The reaction of both the GMC and the Inquiry appears disproportionate if it were only about a relatively small number of deaths following surgery for a complex operation that carried a substantial risk to the patient whoever performed it at that time. An important revelation was the failure to be open about the results; openness might well have allowed the problem to be corrected before it reached the level of catastrophe.

From complex congenital surgery to all results: why the net was cast wider

There is another aspect of Bristol that may assist a better understanding of how a local problem of poor results in complex surgery on babies resulted in a directive to publish mortality figures for routine coronary surgery in adults, and to name the surgeons. In 1997, an Independent Review of Adult Cardiac Surgery was commissioned by The Bristol Royal Infirmary through the Royal College of Surgeons of England.[13] An analysis was made of all adult cardiac surgery from January 1993 to the end of September 1995 – a total of over 2500 cases. The notes were searched by a highly experienced data extractor, 6% were repeated by a second independent data extractor, and the data were 99.7% complete for all the elements required for the Parsonnet risk scoring system prevalent at the time.[14,15] At the outset, there was an explicit agreement that, whatever the findings, they would be disseminated and learned from. In the event, when the code was broken, an outlying surgeon was asked to stop operating. The results were based on large numbers for a single operation with a robust risk adjustment in place, so the statistical conclusions were credible.* A belief that poor results could be attributed to an adverse case mix was refuted. Strangely, adult results were not within the scope of the Bristol Inquiry and were never widely publicized. But they were known. If there had been openness about performance in the much larger-volume coronary surgery, the problem might have been faced and resolved.

Data help institutional development

There is a long tradition of data collection in cardiac surgery. Heart–lung machines were expensive, so start-up costs were high and colleagues were dubious about the merits of cardiac surgery. Surgeons who began to have good results naturally wanted to justify the risk they had taken. They were also campaigning for more resources. Twenty years ago in the *BMJ*, the Society of Cardiothoracic Surgeons of Great Britain and Ireland published data from its cardiac surgical register (Figure 10.2).[16] This initiative was driven by surgeons. Figures for 1977–82 showed wide variation in provision of coronary operations – from 14 per million of the population in southwest England to 200 per million in the London area. The northwest and Mersey were well down at 50 per million. Reporting was by hospital (not surgeon) and the hospital's identity was deliberately concealed before collation. It is generally believed (and in fact is beyond doubt) that this was part of a drive towards equitable distribution of care and a plan for delivery according to patients' needs, not professionals' enthusiasms. The National Service Framework was a long time in germinating and coming to fruition, but this was one of the seeds. It had nothing to do with naming and shaming.

Outcome data inform personal reflection

Apart from campaigning for resources, a secondary purpose emerged – to improve surgical standards. The UK Cardiac Surgery Register was a professional initiative started years before the buzzwords 'clinical audit', 'the quality agenda' and 'clinical governance' were coined, and a very long time

---

* It seems incongruous that the surgeon with the poorest results in the much more commonplace adult coronary surgery was doing the technically most exacting paediatric surgery.

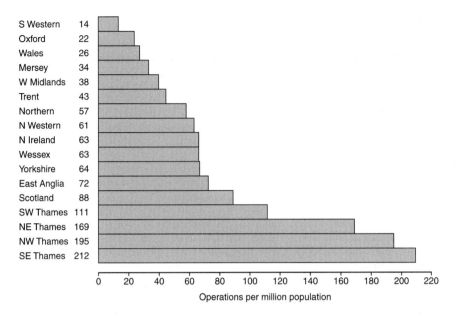

S Western	14
Oxford	22
Wales	26
Mersey	34
W Midlands	38
Trent	43
Northern	57
N Western	61
N Ireland	63
Wessex	63
Yorkshire	64
East Anglia	72
Scotland	88
SW Thames	111
NE Thames	169
NW Thames	195
SE Thames	212

Operations per million population

FIGURE 10.2 Histogram showing average annual number of operations for ischaemic heart disease per million population for each health region during 1977–82. (English TA *et al*, *BMJ* 1984; **289:** 1205–8. Amended with permission from the BMJ Publishing Group.)

before the National Health Service fell in love with organizations with acronyms such as CHI (Commission for Health Improvement) and NICE (National Institute for Clinical Excellence). The objectives of the founding fathers of the UK Register were clear. It was possible for us all to see the results that were being achieved nationally and whether results in our own unit were about the same, better or worse, without the need for anyone to be pilloried.

Simply knowing where one sits in the spread of results allows a team with poorer performance to know who gets the best results, to find out why, and to seek to emulate them. Gawande[1] describes that process for cystic fibrosis. There is a landmark example for the arterial switch operation when a small cluster of failures was addressed by learning from the practice of a unit with the best results.[8] Explicit external comparison was used constructively in both instances. The spirit of the UK Cardiac Surgery Register was to know your own data and compare it with the anonymized data of others.

Just as not all the thoracic surgeons of the 1950s made the successful transition to the new 'open heart' surgery, not all of the new breed of cardiac surgeons of the 1960s and 1970s performing successful heart valve surgery took to the more technically demanding coronary surgery. In the 1980s, it became much less acceptable to do a few congenital operations in children among a largely adult practice. This evolution was influenced by data in the UK Cardiac Register Annual Reports. Confidentiality was regarded as paramount, but it is a close relative of concealment. There were instances where that process of introspection failed and surgeons had to be told to stop. Bristol is by far the most publicized example. The Society of Cardiothoracic Surgeons' data given and kept under a promise of confidentiality and anonymity, were taken to Bristol under a subpoena.

Journals publish data: Do they not set the standard?

A dataset to be used for comparison is only useful if figures are known for all units. There will always be a reporting bias if publication is voluntary. Also, the preferred data can be presented in a journal, in a format that puts the best gloss on the results. To be useful as a monitoring standard, all units must provide equivalent information on all cases. It is highly probable that for both coronary surgery and cystic fibrosis, those at the better end of a performance are more likely to publish results voluntarily.

In practice, in the absence of more appropriate data, journal publications are used and cited in court as *de facto* standards. This is unfortunate because it is not reasonable to expect all surgeons to match the performance of those exemplary individuals whose series are so good that they seek to publish them. Controlled trials are also misleading because they are on highly selected populations and do not reflect the breadth of clinical practice.

Registry data are more appropriate for fair comparisons

A factual record of what actually happens in terms of outcomes, including outcomes for jobbing surgeons as well as the great and the good, is the yardstick. The acquisition and publication of data on outcomes across all centres and surgeons is essential, but at the time of writing, a substantial number of units are unable to comply with Mr Milburn's request for data that are 'robust, rigorous and risk-adjusted'.[11] Until they all do, we cannot use them for comparative purposes.

It is worth mentioning in passing that it is in surgeons' self-interest and self-protection that data on all outcomes likely to be used for comparison are in the public domain, anonymized or not. Suspensions and investigations of individual performance are painful processes not without the dangers of finger-pointing and the blood lust of the witch-hunt. A surgeon can quite rightly feel aggrieved when facing disciplinary action if the only 'factual' evidence of inadequate performance stems from two or three published articles of doubtful provenance, possibly cherry-picked from the literature, which in any case has a cherry-picking publication bias of its own.

Will patients use outcome data to inform choice?

When we are given information on outcomes, what can patients do with the information? Gawande[1] explores the choices for Annie's folks, the cystic fibrosis family, when they discover that their local children's hospital, while taking excellent care of them in every way they could discern, was actually well below average. Should they travel to the unit at the top of the league table? Can patients realistically choose to move their care to another centre on the basis of outcome data? In some instances yes, but in many the choices are few and obstacles to moving are high, so the information may not be of direct help to the individual with burns, a myocardial infarct or lung cancer. At the time of the illness, they may have to go to where care is on offer. It is for the service to address any unevenness discovered. Just as for air travel, the public want to trust the whole process. To post the pilots' names on the ticket, with the implied message that the decision is down to the passenger, does little to address the real issues of safety and institutional accountability. To put outcome figures in the public domain, whether for cystic fibrosis or coronary surgery, with no considered purpose in mind may give many sick people (Annie for example) impossible choices and added anxiety.

Naming surgeons

Implicit in the drive to name the surgeon is the belief that the surgeon is the main determinant of survival.

Is the surgeon individually the most important component of outcome?

Is it self-evident that hospital death after coronary surgery is an outcome dependent on the surgeon, or is this a wrong assumption? Risk factors that depend on the patient (age, previous infarction, diabetes, hypertension and renal failure) must be adjusted for, but that having been done, it can be argued that the surgeon is a key determinant. Let us consider what most deaths are caused by. The major perioperative factors are myocardial function and bleeding. More specifically, they are the effectiveness of the grafts in delivering blood to the previously ischaemic myocardium, protection of the myocardium from ischaemia while the grafts are being fashioned, and ensuring the suture lines are all blood-tight at completion. These are three factors are dependent on the surgeon. Furthermore, the surgeon actually restores the heart to a safer and better functional state. No other member of the team can do that.

On the contrary, anyone can kill the patient. An anaesthetist who is heavy-handed with the drugs, or fails to respond promptly and appropriately to changes in the patient's state, gives the surgeon a very different experience compared with the cool 'steady hand on the tiller' that is much appreciated by the surgeon. An ITU nurse might give a lethal bolus of potassium. Those accidents apart, and in the majority of instances, survival after a heart operation is heavily dependent on the operator's skill and judgement.

In contrast, consider cystic fibrosis. Variation in survival between centres, although large,[1] cannot be related to a single intervention, or a single individual, but to the efforts of a multidisciplinary team over the lifetime of the patient.

Let us take for argument that these two – technique-dependent cardiac operations and the managements of cystic fibrosis – are end-markers of a number of clinical processes and procedures. At the one end, we might place coronary surgery, where an individual's performance at a single event in time is the largest single determinant. Survival after cancer surgery is less clearly dependent on the individual operator. When we perform major cancer surgery on the lung, bowel, oesophagus or pelvic organs, we are usually dealing with older people with a range of comorbidities. Take, for example, pneumonectomy – an operation with a hospital mortality rate of 10–15%.[17,18] Contrast that with coronary artery bypass graft (CABG) mortality rates, which are around 2%. Unlike a coronary operation, where the procedure improves the heart and equips patients better to survive, lung resection inevitably takes away function. Most candidates are ageing lifelong smokers, and a major determinant is the patient. The important outcome is cure from lung cancer, not just short-term survival,[19] and in any case it would be wrong to make judgements for a patient that are aimed at protecting the operator's figures.[20] Survival is determined by factors in perioperative care that probably outweigh those attributable to variations in the technical skill of the specialized surgeons involved.

Pneumonectomy sits somewhere in the middle ground between a single, skill-dependent event such as a coronary operation and the lifelong management of cystic fibrosis by a team. In an attempt to analyse these factors, the Association of Cardiothoracic Anaesthetists is collecting data during 2005 to give insight into variations in case selection, work-up, intraoperative management and postoperative care of pneumonectomy.

In the process of cancer care, there is a sequence that more or less goes like this:

1. A suspicion of cancer arises.
2. The suspicion is supported by imaging of one sort or another.

3. The diagnosis is confirmed by biopsy.
4. A clinical estimate is made of the options for treatment, and surgery may be precluded at this stage.
5. If staging-dependent treatment is considered, further tests, scans and biopsies are performed.
6. A view is taken by a multidisciplinary team as to which treatment combination will be used.
7. If the cancer is staged as amenable to surgery, more detailed fitness evaluation is performed.
8. If deemed fit for surgery, an anaesthetist uses skills to have the patient asleep and pain-free, intubated and suitably monitored.
9. The surgeon operates.
10. The patient is nursed to recovery.

The surgeon is only a part of that process.

Naming surgeons may be damaging for patients

Attributing outcome to individual surgeons within a service may not be in the interest of patients. There are detrimental effects. In surgery for any life-threatening conditions, it is often the very patients who have the most to gain in terms of added life-years and quality who face the highest perioperative risk of death. In the case of coronary surgery, for example, if a surgeon has had a death in the previous 10 patients, the pressure is on to avoid any deaths in the next 40 to achieve 98% survival – the average for published data.

In cancer surgery, the patient may face certain death from the condition. What operative risk would be acceptable to the patient? Case selection to protect mortality figures is not in the patient's interest. Risk adjustment and use of confidence intervals should prevent incorrect inferences being drawn about performance, but a surgeon might simply become selective.

Another consideration is that if a patient is irretrievable – and this may be unrelated to the operation itself – the surgeon may continue to strive unrealistically for survival in the interests of protecting figures. This happens now. The decision should be what is in the patient's overall best interests and should take into consideration the resource implications for other patients. Blocked ITU beds mean cancelled surgery.

Naming surgeons will be damaging for surgeons

So far, we have only considered the downside for patients. What about for surgeons? Once we acknowledge that, no matter how much we improve our average, the bell distribution curve is not going to go away, we are left with all sorts of questions. Gawande[1] asks:

- Will being in the bottom half be used against doctors in lawsuits?
- Will we be expected to tell our patients how we score?
- Will our patients leave us?
- Will those at the bottom be paid less than those at the top?

He answers 'yes' to all of these questions. If any of these adverse outcomes for the surgeon occur on the basis of unreliable, inaccurate or non-risk-adjusted data, surgeons would be harmed unfairly. Nor is this of help to the public if expensively trained and capable surgeons are lost to the service.

Measures of the objective might be more useful than naming surgeons

Knowledge of the hospital's overall care process and outcomes would be more in the patients' interests than naming surgeons. For example, ischaemic heart disease can be managed medically, by angioplasty or by surgery. There are ways of shifting the risk – with a tendency for the highest-risk cases to arrive on the surgeon's operating table.

Ischaemic heart disease management has an escalation series of treatments. Medical management (i.e. tablets and pills) is the first line. If that is not solving the problem, the cardiologist will do angiography and see if the condition is amenable to or preferably managed by a percutaneous intervention. If not, referral to surgery is the next course of action. Progression through this sequence may be rapid (within hours) or take years, but at each transition, most judgements are made by the physicians and some (but relatively few) by the patient. What the patient deserves is that the decisions be well made, not just that the procedures be well done. Auditing one sector without looking at the overall outcomes clearly creates an opportunity for the risk to be shifted for various reasons. This can go in both directions. Refusing to operate on high-risk cases disadvantages the patient, but also persevering with conservative management until the risks are high may miss the opportunity for a good outcome. Ideally, if one could do it, decisions should be audited as well as events, and the service should be considered as a whole. Knowing only the surgeons' operative mortality rates may be something of a red herring when selecting appropriate treatment options.

What can we learn from civil aviation?

It is quite common now for symposia on surgical teams and errors to include a speaker from the aviation industry. They know about these things. They have well-rehearsed safety procedures and methods of deconstructing what went wrong. They have a special problem that we do not share. Individual pilots' crash statistics probably never include a series amenable to statistical analysis; for critical failure, $N=1$ so 'near-misses' are the only adverse outcome amenable to analysis. While we recognize that we have a lot to learn from their processes, what we do know for certain is that we, the passengers, never see named pilots' records of 'near-misses' publicized when we choose which airline to fly with or indeed whether to take that particular flight. They promise us a safe flight, which includes the maintenance of the plane and its navigation. They do not leave it up to us to base our decision to fly on the name of the captain rostered that day. There may be good reasons why airlines do not tell us the flying record of the pilot, which may include some of the arguments given above, but it does not mean that they do not know.

Are mortality rates an informative measure of quality?

In many instances, it would be sensible to broaden the outcome reported. Freedom from stroke may depend on who does the carotid endarterectomy, continence might depend on who does the rectal excision, and years of pain-free walking might depend on who replaces the joint. For many procedures, death is rare and should never happen – ENT surgery in children for example. A zero mortality rate may be compatible with both a distinguished career of excellent surgery and a lifetime of abysmal performance.

One should really consider spreading the net even wider. Consider an analogy between surgical processes and industry. A factory owner concerned with the quality of the widgets that his factory produces does not stand at the factory gate and monitor the quality of what is shipped out, with the intention of closing the factory down or sacking the operations manager if quality slips. That is clearly stupid, yet such a focus on counting what is most easily countable is perhaps a consequence of Bristol.

Why is it stupid to stand at the factory gate and count the substandard widgets? In the real world of manufacturing, one takes a systems view. Factories can be noisy, dirty and quite unpleasant environments, yet, by and large, they are very well ordered. There are many interacting processes that go on: raw materials are ordered, delivered and stored. They are transported to machines, processed and turned into widget components. These are then assembled, tested and then adjusted. They are stamped, packaged and packed into cartons. All these processes interact, and if there are quality problems then that is where they occur, not at the factory gate. Any good production manager knows that you make sure the individual processes all operate well.

From an operational research perspective, hospitals are not really different from factories. While the hospital is there to serve patients, fragile humans with feelings and dignity, taking a dispassionate view, one can also regard patients as widgets being 'processed' as they pass through different phases of their care pathway as illustrated in Figure 10.3. Building on this mechanistic view of the surgical process, one can also consider the associated healthcare teams that the patient encounters during the course of their care. A simplistic example of this is illustrated in Figure 10.4.

Taking this systems view immediately shifts the focus from 'factory gate' monitoring. The patient's care involves a concatenation of input from many different care teams, and careful handover between such teams. Problems occur when the working of the overall team is disrupted – not necessarily under the surgeon's scalpel. True, knives are very dangerous, but so too are dirty wards, lost notes and misdiagnoses on referral. It is the system, not the individual, that should be scrutinized.

Mindless data collection

We turn now to a central difficulty associated with publishing individual surgical data. How does one avoid the data being misinterpreted? Certainly, Bristol 'was awash with data',[1] however this is not to say that it was awash

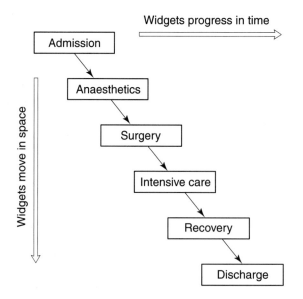

FIGURE 10.3 A simplistic representation of the surgical healthcare process viewed from a systems perspective.

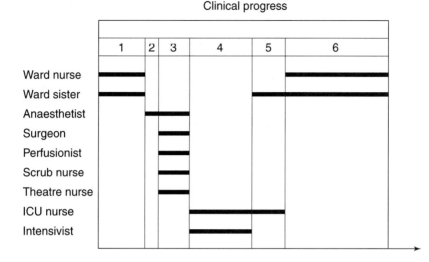

FIGURE 10.4 Contacts between the widget (patient) and processes (care team).

with useful information. It is a common misconception that these two notions are synonymous, yet how many times have eager young researchers, with laptops full of numbers collected over many months, knocked on the door of a statistical advisor hoping to be told the magic words that will somehow release the truth that must surely be there. Alas, all too often, data are just numbers and they do not tell us very much.

Difficult statistical issues

Even in the case of Bristol, with the cartons of data assembled, an expert statistical team faced enormous difficulties interpreting what the numbers meant. Even the simplest questions such as 'was mortality at Bristol higher than anywhere else?' required extraordinary complex analysis and there was a need to appeal to some techniques that were not in standard statistics books.[21] What is the general public, or indeed the majority of the surgical profession, expected to learn from published mortality data when in general they have neither the skills in interpreting complex data nor an awareness of potential pitfalls of statistical analysis that can delude the unwary.[22]

What are 99.99% confidence intervals about?

We give an example. The cardiac surgeons of the SCTS decided to publish data with 99.99% confidence intervals:[12]

It is reasonable that the threshold should be considerably higher when risk adjustment is not used than when it is. So how has the society set the limits? In industry, 99.9% confidence limits (3 SD) are commonly used for quality control processes for manufacturing, where there is control of raw materials. Sadly, this level of standardization does not hold for cardiac surgery patients, who can be very heterogeneous. So the limits were widened to 99.99% (4 SD) to take this additional, inherent variation into consideration. The society proposes to use these limits as its basis for publication of individual surgeons' results. So, for the purposes of safety, it will consider that any surgeon whose mortality is within 99.99% (4 SD) over an aggregated three-year period will have met transparent and defined standards.

The effect of this 'standard' is that a surgeon whose competence is actually within the range of normal would fall outside these confidence intervals only once in 10 000 similar runs of cases. The other side of the coin is that, by this yardstick, a surgeon with questionable performance would not come to light for many years. Is that what Kennedy and Millburn had in mind? To understand what is happening here, consider the problem of setting the sensitivity on an alarm. When we set a security system to detect intruders, we make choices about the triggering sensitivity of various devices. If we set the system very sensitively, every stray cat, passing fire engine or gust of wind will trigger it. Conversely, if it is so robust that nothing short of a man with a sledgehammer laying into the front door will produce a response, it fails as an early-warning system. This latter case is akin to the 99.99% confidence intervals. The surgical carnage required to trigger an alarm at that threshold would be truly dreadful.

Setting the threshold lower would mean in the case of the burglar alarm that an innocent bystander might fall under suspicion or several entirely satisfactory surgeons suffer a bad time at the hands of their medical directors and the press, only to be exonerated later.

How long is a bad run?

There are occasions when the statistical evidence seems compelling that something is amiss, yet this might arise purely as a statistical artefact. For example, in the case of operations that are performed relatively infrequently, publishing annual mortality rates and making judgments based on these is equivalent to inference based on relatively short runs of success or failure. This poses rather difficult methodological problems.[23] Can one ever be certain that a run of poor outcomes truly reflects an unacceptably high mortality risk? The alternative is that it might be a chance occurrence, particularly if the number of cases in the run is small.

One can draw an analogy with coin tossing. If one tossed a coin 4 times, it would not be very surprising if it were to land showing heads 3 out of the 4 times. If the coin toss were perfectly fair, this would occur for 25% of such sequences. On the other hand, if the first time one tossed a coin 8 times, it came up heads 7 times, one might justifiably be suspicious (but not certain) that it was biased, since the probability of this happening is approximately 3%. However, if one were to toss a perfectly fair coin 300 times, the chances of having a run of 8 tosses with 7 heads at some time during the whole sequence is about 98% – a virtual certainty. Such analysis is perhaps somewhat counterintuitive to non-mathematicians, yet it has potentially serious consequences for the surgical profession.

Inescapably, given any list of numbers, one of them must be highest. Thus, if a 'league table' is published for named surgeons, one unfortunate individual will have the highest mortality rate. Equally, the more operations a surgeon performs, the more likely it is that a short-term run of apparent poor outcome will occur.

We are thus faced with a serious dilemma. On the one hand, we need to set our security alarm system so that it detects a miscreant somewhat less threatening than a sledgehammer-wielding maniac. On the other hand, it would be a comfort if the majority of surgeons could embark on their careers without knowing that there was a reasonable chance that they would be suspended, and perhaps pilloried in the press, before a well-earned retirement. How best can the middle ground be found? That is a challenge for this era of surgical performance monitoring.

Onora O'Neill, in her Reith Lectures, warned of dangers:[24]

'Perhaps the culture of accountability that we are relentlessly building for ourselves actually damages trust rather than supports it. Plants don't flourish when we pull them up too often to check how their roots are growing.'

References

1. Gawande A. The bell curve. What happens when patients find out how good their doctors really are? *The New Yorker* 6 December 2004.
2. Geddes DM. Cystic fibrosis: epidemiology and pathogenesis. In: Brewis RAL, Corrin B, Geddes DM, Gibson GJ (eds). *Respiratory Medicine*. London: WB Saunders, 1995: 1317–29.
3. Corner EM. *St Thomas' Hospital Reports*, 1900.
4. Hey Groves EW. A plea for a uniform registration of operation results. *BMJ* 1908; **ii**: 1008–9.
5. Fox R, Swazey J. The heart transplant moratorium. In: *The Courage to Fail. A social view of organ transplants and dialysis*. London, Chicago: University of Chicago Press, 1974. 60–83.

6. Cutler EC, Beck CS. Present status of surgical procedures in chronic valvular disease of the heart; final report of all surgical cases. *Arch Surg* 1929; **18**: 402–16.
7. Treasure T, Hollman A. The surgery of mitral stenosis 1898–1948: Why did it take 50 years to establish mitral valvotomy? *Ann R Coll Surg Engl* 1995; **77**: 145–51.
8. de Leval MR, Francois K, Bull C *et al*. Analysis of a cluster of surgical failures. Application to a series of neonatal arterial switch operations. *J Thorac Cardiovasc Surg* 1994; **107**: 914–23.
9. Treasure T. A brief history of evidence. In: Treasure T *et al* (eds). *The Evidence for Cardiothoracic Surgery*. Shrewsbury, UK: tfm Publishing 2005: 5–16.
10. Hammond P. Private Eye. http://www.bristol-inquiry.org.uk/final_report/annex_a/chapter_27_6.htm (9), 3–9. 1–3–2005.
11. Bristol Royal Infirmary Inquiry: www.publications.parliament.uk/pa/cm200102/cmhansrd/vo010718/debtext/10718–04.htm, 2005.
12. Keogh B, Spiegelhalter D, Bailey A *et al*. The legacy of Bristol: public disclosure of individual surgeons' results. *BMJ* 2004; **329**: 450–4.
13. Treasure T, Taylor K, Black N. *Independent Review of Adult Cardiac Surgery*. United Bristol Healthcare Trust, 1997.
14. Parsonnet V, Dean D, Bernstein AD. A method of uniform stratification of risk for evaluating the results of surgery in acquired adult heart disease. *Circulation* 1989; **79**: I3–12.
15. Nashef SA, Carey F, Silcock MM *et al*. Risk stratification for open heart surgery: trial of the Parsonnet system in a British hospital. *BMJ* 1992; **305**: 1066–7.
16. English TA, Bailey AR, Dark JF, Williams WG. The UK cardiac surgical register, 1977–82. *BMJ* 1984; **289**: 1205–8.
17. Birkmeyer JD, Siewers AE, Finlayson EV *et al*. Hospital volume and surgical mortality in the United States. *N Engl J Med* 2002; **346**: 1128–37.
18. Birkmeyer JD, Stukel TA, Siewers AE *et al*. Surgeon volume and operative mortality in the United States. *N Engl J Med* 2003; **349**: 2117–27.
19. Treasure T, Utley M, Bailey A. Assessment of whether in-hospital mortality for lobectomy is a useful standard for the quality of lung cancer surgery: retrospective study. *BMJ* 2003; **327**: 73.
20. Treasure T. Whose lung is it anyway? *Thorax* 2002; **57**: 3–4.
21. Gallivan S. Assessing mortality rates from dubious data – when to stop doing statistics and start doing mathematics. *Health Care Management Science* [In press].
22. Huff D. How to lie with statistics. New York: W. W. Norton & Co. 1993.
23. Gallivan S. How likely is it that a run of poor outcomes is unlikely: *Eur J of Operational Research* 2003; **1:** 46–52.
24. O'Neill O. *A Question of Trust: the BBC Reith Lectures 2002*. Cambridge: Cambridge University Press, 2002.

11

Professional self-regulation, revalidation, poor performance and clinical governance

David Hatch

Patients and doctors have a common interest in effective medical professionalism,[1] and the need for doctors to adhere to contemporary professional standards has been recognized since the Hippocratic oath was first stated in the 5th century BC. One of the main reasons for the establishment of the early professional societies, and later the Royal Colleges, was the acknowledged need to protect patients from quackery by setting professional standards and ensuring their maintenance by a system of self-regulation. The Society of Apothecaries established an organized system of education, qualification and registration in 1815, and the need for medical practice to be supported by a regulatory body with statutory disciplinary powers was recognized by the establishment of the General Medical Council (GMC) in 1858. However, until as recently as 1980, the GMC Disciplinary Committee was limited to the consideration of allegations of *infamous conduct*, subsequently known as *serious professional misconduct*. Virtually all the cases heard by this committee related to allegations of criminal behaviour by doctors or serious abuse of the doctor/patient relationship, and the GMC played virtually no role in relation to doctors whose professional clinical standards of care were unsatisfactory unless they amounted to criminal negligence. The GMC has now made the professional standards required of doctors on the Medical Register more explicit by the publication of the booklet *Good Medical Practice*.[2] Some doctors have been under the misapprehension that this is a statement of the ideals to which doctors should aspire rather than a guide to the basic principles of competence, care and conduct expected of all doctors by the profession. The 2001 edition makes it clear that serious or persistent failure to meet the standards in the booklet may put a doctor's registration at risk.

In 1980, following the successful Sick Doctor Scheme introduced by the Association of Anaesthetists of Great Britain and Ireland, the GMC introduced its Health Procedures designed to deal with doctors whose performance was seriously affected by their own state of health. Designed primarily to protect the public by either applying conditions to or suspending the doctor's registration, these procedures also allowed for the doctor found to be suffering from *seriously impaired health* to receive remedial treatment and rehabilitation. In 1997, the GMC introduced its performance procedures under which doctors whose clinical performance was found to be *seriously deficient* following a comprehensive assessment of their clinical practice could also have their registration affected. These procedures also allowed the doctor to be given an opportunity for retraining where this is deemed to be realistic, although at present the opportunities for retraining are extremely limited.

The GMC has recognized for some time that dysfunction in a doctor's practice may be due to a combination of conduct, health and performance issues. Under its new rules, introduced on 1 November 2004, all of these matters may be considered by a single committee, who will determine whether there is a reasonable prospect of proving that a doctor's fitness to practise is impaired to a degree that warrants action on registration.

The Royal Colleges have developed excellent training programmes leading to speciality recognition within each field, but have devoted far less time to lifelong learning, continuing education and professional development (CPD). The GMC has now issued guidance to support both formal and informal CPD.[3] The limitations of voluntary unstructured continuing medical education undertaken by the committed majority and avoided by those who may be in most need of it are being addressed.

Despite these and other continuing initiatives by the profession, including the increase in the GMC's non-medical membership from 10% to 40% over the last ten years, together with the commitment of most individual doctors to the maintenance of high standards of practice, more needs to be done. Recent high-profile examples of doctors whose professional standards have been seriously deficient have been given extensive coverage by the news media. The fact that these doctors have in some cases been allowed to practise for several years despite their serious deficiencies being known to close colleagues has been a source of justifiable concern to both the Government and the public. Although the most recent surveys suggest that public confidence in doctors remains high, the ability of the profession to regulate itself in a way that protects patients from dangerous members of the profession has been increasingly questioned.

Revalidation

The purpose of revalidation is to ensure that patients can have confidence that doctors are competent and abide by high ethical standards. It aims at encouraging all doctors to reflect on their work, using evidence from their own practice gathered through audit and in other ways. Members of the public understandably expect the Medical Register to indicate those doctors who are currently fit to practise, and many are surprised to learn that this has not been the case. Until recently, there has been no mechanism for assessing the conduct, health or performance of any doctor on the Medical Register unless allegations of serious deficiency against them are reported to the GMC. The Register's Principal List thus only provides a list of names of people who have at some time, possibly many decades ago, passed an accepted qualifying examination and satisfactorily completed a period of provisional or temporary registration and against whom nothing adverse is known by the GMC. Similarly, many doctors are on the Specialist Register by virtue of their consultant status, which may have been obtained many years ago.

This is no longer adequate to satisfy public demand for assurances that doctors remain capable and safe throughout their practising lives.[4] Despite the explicit professional obligation in *Good Medical Practice* for doctors to act quickly to protect patients when a colleague may not be fit to practise, there is still a degree of reluctance among some doctors to 'blow the whistle' in this situation. It is therefore clear that any system that relies solely on reporting of poor practice is unlikely to be sufficient in the long term to maintain public confidence in the profession. In addition, many doctors would welcome the opportunity to demonstrate that they are giving good medical care, and to be helped to correct any weaknesses promptly in a supportive environment.

The GMC has therefore resolved that continued registration should be linked with regular active demonstration by all registered doctors that they remain fit to practise and up to date in their chosen field. There is, however, no evidence that periodic re-certification of credentials by some form of examination bears any relation to clinical performance, so the GMC has decided to adopt a performance-based system, which has become known as revalidation.

The introduction of an effective and simple system of revalidation will be critical in ensuring that all doctors subject their practices to regular review and will be a touchstone of credibility for the GMC. All doctors will be required to keep a folder of evidence, drawn from their own medical practice, to demonstrate that they have been practising in accordance with the standards of competence, care and conduct set out in *Good Medical Practice*. These include not only the provision of good clinical care and the professional obligation upon doctors to keep up to date, but also relationships with patients and colleagues, teaching and training, probity and health. While many of these attributes are generic, most Royal Colleges and specialist associations have published guidance on how the principles in the guidance apply in the particular practice circumstances of their members.

In future, the rights and privileges currently granted to doctors who are registered with the GMC will become dependent upon the doctor holding a licence to practise. Doctors will be required to satisfy the GMC on a regular basis, every five years, that they are up to date and fit to practise. This process of revalidation will be a condition of a doctor's continued licensure with the GMC. When they receive their first licence, doctors will be advised of the submission year during which they will first be required to undergo revalidation. The first submissions were to be required in the year July 2005–June 2006, followed by a rolling programme related to the penultimate digit of the doctor's GMC number (Table 11.1). However, Dame Janet Smith, in the Fifth Report of the Shipman Enquiry,[5] has expressed her concern about the ability of the GMC's revalidation proposals to demonstrate that doctors are up to date and fit to practise. Following the publication of this Report in December 2004, the GMC and Department of Health have expressed the wish to consider their response to the whole report rather than implement changes piecemeal, and to review all its implications for licensing and revalidation. The Chief Medical Officer will lead a review, which will include the role of NHS appraisal and cover the GMC's arrangements for examining a doctor's fitness to practise within the revalidation process. As a result, the intended launch of revalidation has been postponed.

Doctors who, through retirement, career breaks, overseas practice or other reason, decide not to hold a licence to practise, whether or not they remain on the GMC register, will no longer be able to exercise any of the privileges formerly conferred on them by registration, including prescribing. However, the lack of a licence will not prevent them from undertaking Good Samaritan acts or work for which registration is not needed, such as signing passport

TABLE 11.1 The GMC's proposed submission years for doctors to provide the evidence for revalidation of their licence to practise[a]

Penultimate digit of the doctor's GMC registration number	Submission Year
0	July 2005–June 2006
1 and 6	July 2006–June 2007
2 and 7	July 2007–June 2008
3 and 8	July 2008–June 2009
4, 5 and 9	July 2009–June 2010

[a] Subsequently postponed pending consideration of the implications of the Shipman Inquiry.

photographs. The GMC will expect doctors, whether or not holding a licence or registered, to offer assistance in an emergency. *Good Medical Practice* says: 'In an emergency, wherever it may arise, you must offer anyone at risk the treatment you could reasonably be expected to provide.' Medical defence organizations may have different arrangements for providing indemnity cover depending on whether a doctor holds a licence or registration only. Unlicenced doctors should talk to their medical defence organizations about their indemnity for clinical negligence claims arising from Good Samaritan acts.

Although failure to participate in revalidation will ultimately lead to loss of a doctor's licence to practise, doctors who provide the evidence described above will not face the threat of any new GMC disciplinary procedures. Where revalidation reveals serious problems that have not been satisfactorily resolved locally, the doctor will be treated in the same way as those referred to the GMC by a complainant. The doctor's right to practise will only be affected if a GMC Fitness to Practise Panel finds the doctor's fitness to practice is impaired to a degree that warrants action on registration. Otherwise, their licence will be revalidated. It should be remembered, however, that as part of the recent reform of its fitness-to-practise procedures, the GMC has now developed the concept of 'warnings'. A warning may be given when there has been a significant departure from *Good Medical Practice* that is not so serious as to justify action on a doctor's registration but requires action from the GMC in the interests of maintaining good professional standards and public confidence in the profession. Warnings will remain on a doctor's record for five years and will be disclosable to enquirers. The GMC will want to see evidence that the problems that gave rise to the warning have been addressed by the time of the doctor's next revalidation.

On 1 October 1999, there were 193 366 doctors on the register, of whom 36 199 were on the specialist register. Registered doctors work in a wide variety of chosen fields, while, for a variety of different reasons, some do not practise at all and may opt to move to a register of unvalidated doctors. Some doctors are registered in more than one specialty and not all are members of Royal Colleges, faculties or specialist associations. The majority of doctors in active clinical practice in the UK work in some capacity within the NHS at various grades and in various specialities. The NHS can be split roughly into two main areas: hospital practice and general practice. The former category includes consultants, non-consultant career-grade doctors, clinical assistants, doctors in training, and others in Trust doctor and similar grades. The latter category contains GP principals and non-principals, and GP registrars. There are also doctors employed within the Department of Health, the NHS Executive, Health Authorities, Boards and Trusts who may not be engaged in the direct clinical care of patients. This group includes doctors employed in public health medicine and some medical directors. In addition to the NHS, there are a number of other public sector areas in which doctors work, such as the prison service and armed forces. There are also many doctors who work outside the NHS, for example those engaged in full-time private medical practice, occupational health doctors in private companies, doctors employed by the pharmaceutical and other industries, and ships' doctors. Some doctors undertake clinical work for more than one organization at the same time or may work independently outside their main area of employment. Locum doctors perform an extremely valuable function and work in most areas of medical practice. A recent audit commission report on locum doctors states that on a typical day there are around 3500 doctors working as locums in England and Wales. Some doctors are only engaged in active medical practice on a part-time basis, and where they practise only intermittently it may be difficult for them to provide evidence of their fitness to practise. Others are not in active clinical practice but may require continued registration, such as some who hold teaching posts, those retained by firms of solicitors to provide medico-legal reports, those employed in medico-political work or those holding high national office such as the President of the GMC and the four Chief Medical Officers. A separate issue is raised by those doctors who may be employed for a time in primary administrative capacities but who may wish to return to medical practice at a later date, for example undergraduate or postgraduate deans. Of the 191 682 doctors on the principal list in October 1999, 165 607 had registered addresses in the UK and 26 075 had registered addresses elsewhere. It does not necessarily follow that a registered address in the UK signifies that a doctor works in the UK or that an address abroad means that a doctor lives and works abroad. Some doctors choose for a variety of reasons to take a career break of variable duration, after which they may wish to return to active clinical practice. It is not clear how many doctors on the register have retired from medical practice, and at present there is no record of date of birth on the register. On the assumption that the majority of medical practitioners qualify at the age of 25, deducting 25 from the year of qualification suggests that approximately 30 000 registered doctors are over the age of 70. There is no available information to indicate how many of these doctors are involved in any form of clinical practice or exercising any of the privileges of registration. Anecdotal evidence suggests that retired doctors not infrequently prescribe for family and friends.

It is clear from the above analysis that the development of revalidation systems for all categories of doctors is not going to be an easy task. In addressing this problem, the GMC has decided that revalidation should be based as far as possible on existing and proposed local quality arrangements. Some of these are outlined below.

Doctors practising in the UK primarily in the NHS or other GMC-approved environments

The 'GMC-approved environment' is an important concept in the system of licensing and revalidation. A GMC-approved environment will be regarded as a practice setting in the UK, whether operating in the NHS or elsewhere, that is subject to systems that provide:

- clear lines of responsibility for the overall quality of care
- clear policies aimed at managing risk
- procedures for all professional groups to identify and remedy poor performance
- appropriate supervision arrangements for doctors
- a comprehensive programme of quality improvement activities, such as CPD, guidelines, incident reporting and clinical audit
- an annual appraisal or assessment process, based on the principles of *Good Medical Practice*, for individual practitioners
- quality assurance by an acceptable independent UK-based body such as the Healthcare Commission in England

Most doctors in the NHS and in other GMC-approved environments, including GPs, now undergo regular appraisal. This fulfils the first aim of revalidation – to encourage doctors to reflect upon their work – provided that it is based on evidence derived from their practice and is mapped against the headings of *Good Medical Practice*. For doctors working primarily in such environments, the evidence for revalidation should come from confirmation of their participation in appraisal and certification by an appropriately authorized person that there are no significant unresolved concerns about their fitness to practise. The GMC does not intend to scrutinize every doctor's folder, although a random selection of doctors will be chosen to submit their folder as part of the quality assurance arrangements for revalidation. Chief Executives in NHS Trusts are now accountable to Trust Boards for overseeing the appraisal process and confirming that all doctors have been appraised. They must also ensure that any issues arising out of the appraisals are being properly dealt with and that personal development plans (PDPs) are in place for all. To ensure that appraisal in the NHS is applied consistently and satisfies the GMC's requirements for revalidation, the Department of Health has, in agreement with the British Medical Association (BMA), produced a set of appraisal documentation. Although the purpose of appraisal is formative, it will provide an important opportunity to support revalidation by a review of the doctor's folder, ensuring that the information in it is accurate and sufficient, identifying gaps and difficulties to be addressed, and highlighting any contribution made by environmental factors towards the doctor's performance. Appraisal will provide an opportunity to facilitate or arrange any developmental or remedial action required and agree a personal development plan for the coming year. Doctors undertaking appraisals will, in exceptional circumstances, have, under their professional duties to the GMC, to take appropriate steps to protect patients from dangerously poor performance by the doctor being appraised. In these circumstances, the appraisal should be terminated until the concern has been dealt with by other means. However, in the vast majority of cases, regular annual appraisal will allow a doctor to accumulate the evidence required within the five-year time frame for revalidation and ensure that there are no surprises at the end of this period. Some Royal Colleges and specialist associations are already providing guidance on the nature of the information required for their members in the revalidation folder, helping to define recommended standards for audit and offering help when problems arise. The Joint Committee on Good Practice of the Royal College and Association of Anaesthetists has devised a list of recommended core topics to help anaesthetists target their continuing medical education and professional development.[6] Some Royal Colleges have produced audit 'recipe books' to help their members target their audit activities.[7,8] The Joint Committee on Postgraduate Training in General Practice (JCPTGP) has set out the standards that it expects individual GP trainers to meet and identifies the expected attributes of a training practice. Recognition as a GP trainer is time-limited, and trainers are expected to be willing to have their clinical abilities assessed by their peers. The Royal College of General Practitioners has attempted to define some of the attributes of an excellent and an unacceptable GP,[9] has set up a working group on revalidation and operates a number of different CPD arrangements.

The Private Practice Forum has set out the standards that it expects of all doctors working in private practice.[10] These standards were devised under the auspices of the Academy of Medical Royal Colleges, the BMA, the Independent Healthcare Association and the Association of British Insurers. All private doctors are expected to maintain the current knowledge and skills relevant to their area of speciality and to undertake continuing medical education (CME) in accordance with the standards set down by the appropriate Royal College or faculty. All private doctors are also expected to ensure that they participate in continuous professional development and produce three-year reviews of professional development plans. The management boards of the private hospitals are becoming increasingly careful in checking the professional standards of those doctors to whom they grant admitting rights to their hospitals. Most doctors working in the private sector are also employed in the NHS and will therefore be subject to the appraisal systems described above for hospital doctors. Every private doctor is expected to participate actively in clinical audits, and medical advisory committees should ensure that mandatory audit is carried out, reviewing the results and advising management on any action needed within their hospitals.

The Ministry of Defence is reviewing its practices to ensure that they take account of clinical governance initiatives through liaison with the Department of Health, NHS Executive and GMC. Consultants serving in the armed forces are, like their NHS colleagues, expected to participate in CPD and CME, to develop their skills and keep up to date, and to participate in clinical audit. The JCPTGP is responsible for the approval of all armed services GP training posts and inspects the armed services as part of its accreditation visiting process. All doctors working in the armed forces are subject to an annual appraisal process on the same lines as their non-medical peers. This is undertaken by their line manager with supplementary medical input where necessary.

In a recent NHS Executive and HM Prison Service report,[11] a future strategy for CPD is recommended. It proposes that plans will be in line with present recommendations from the NHS and the Royal Colleges. In the future prison doctors will adopt the quality systems set out in the Department of Health document *A First Class Service*,[12] including appraisal and audit.

The NHS Executive has issued a code of practice on the appointment and employment of locum doctors in an attempt to improve quality control of this group of practitioners. It recommends that a full report on locum doctors should be prepared at the end of each locum period, identifying training needs as well as knowledge, attitudes, relationships and personal qualities of the individual. These reports are likely to form the basis for the locum doctor's revalidation folder, although more work needs to be done to identify mechanisms to enable locum doctors to take part in audit and CPD and to receive the benefits of regular annual appraisal. This group of doctors may well provide the greatest challenge for revalidation.

Doctors in training

Revalidation arrangements for doctors in training should be based as far as possible on existing arrangements for their monitoring, appraisal and assessment. If these arrangements are working properly, the revalidation of a doctor in training who is making satisfactory process either at Senior House Officer, GP registrar or specialist registrar grade should be straightforward. It is the doctor's responsibility to create a professional folder in which to keep all documentation relating to training or continuing professional development, including details of assessments completed and records of appraisals. For the process to be acceptable, however, it must be seen to be underpinned by *Good*

Medical Practice more explicitly than it sometimes is, and the introduction of a lay element into the assessment will need to be considered. Specialist Registrars, whose training is becoming increasingly competency-based, must have at least one appraisal each year to support the Annual RITA Review and GMC revalidation. This appraisal should take place in plenty of time to allow the trainee and trainers to organize any measures agreed at appraisal that may affect the outcome of the RITA Review. A fresh appraisal must precede each RITA. This provides a record of the annual review and of the doctor's progress through the training program and the grade. It is normally completed by the trainee and the postgraduate dean each year. General practice training is delivered within practices by GP trainers accredited by the JCPTGP, which sets the standards for all GP training. However, locum, assistant and deputizing GPs who are eligible to practice by virtue of their acquired rights may have had no training whatsoever in general practice. GP registrars in the UK commencing their training on or after the 30 January 1998 must have passed a test of competence known as summative assessment before they can work unsupervised.

Doctors practising in the UK outside GMC-approved environments

Some doctors practise in the UK primarily in environments where no local certification systems are in place. Many will be able to provide evidence of their participation in appraisal schemes that fulfil the GMC's requirements as outlined above. Such schemes must:

- be based on *Good Medical Practice*
- be based on verifiable evidence
- have produced an agreed personal development plan
- be carried out and signed off by an appraiser who is a licensed medical practitioner

Doctors practising in these environments will not, however, be able to obtain local certification that there are no concerns regarding their fitness to practise. As an alternative to this, the GMC is developing colleague and patient questionnaires for use by these doctors.

Doctors practising overseas

The revalidation requirements for GMC registered doctors practising overseas will depend on their practice situation. Doctors who hold a licence on 1 April

2005 and who work wholly outside the UK in situations where their right to practise in the host country depends upon GMC registration may opt to retain their GMC registration without a licence. If they wish to return to UK practice, even for short-term locum appointments, they must apply in advance to have the licence restored.

The revalidation requirements for doctors practising overseas in GMC-approved environments will be as described above. Doctors practising overseas outside such environments who wish to retain a licence will be required to:

- submit a folder of information drawn from medical practice mapped against *Good Medical Practice*
- provide certificates of good standing from overseas regulatory bodies in each medical jurisdiction in which they have been practising
- provide evidence of health and probity

Doctors with no medical practice

If a licensed doctor who is not engaged in any medical practice from which to draw evidence wishes to seek revalidation, the GMC will expect him or her to provide the results of a suitable objective assessment such as the PLAB or similar test, as well as providing evidence of health and probity.

Further details of the GMC's revalidation requirements and the implications of holding registration only are explained in the GMC's Guidance on Licencing and Revalidation, available from its website (www.gmc-uk.org/revalidation).

Links between revalidation and clinical governance

The concept of clinical governance, now well established in the NHS and developing elsewhere, was first outlined by the Government in a series of publications from 1998 onwards.[12-14] Backed by a statutory duty of quality, its aims were threefold:

- the setting of national standards of care
- monitoring compliance with these standards
- encouragement of lifelong learning, strengthening professional self-regulation and identifying possible lapses in clinical quality at an early stage

The new measures outlined in the consultation document, *Supporting Doctors, Protecting Patients*,[13] are intended to enable NHS trusts and health authorities to take action quickly to detect emerging problems and resolve them quickly and fairly by ensuring that:

- all NHS doctors' practice is monitored to pick up problems early
- poor performance is tackled swiftly
- tough action is taken in response

Hospital doctors and GPs are now required to participate in external clinical audit and take part in an annual appraisal of their performance. Where doctors are suspected of poor practice, Trusts in England are expected to seek advice from an independent and impartial body, the National Clinical Assessment Agency (NCAA), which can, with the agreement of the doctor, undertake a performance assessment, including a behavioural assessment, and may suggest retraining or other remedial needs. If the NCAA feels that the problems cannot be put right locally, it will advise employers accordingly, who can the take necessary action as well as notifying the GMC. The GMC has agreed a memorandum of understanding with the NCAA and is working towards a situation where at least some aspects of a NCAA assessment can be accepted as evidence by the GMC. This would minimize the need for doctors who have been assessed by the NCAA having to undergo a repeat of the assessment by the GMC. It is important, however, that any such disclosure does not undermine a doctor's confidence that information gathered confidentially by the NCAA will be used for remedial rather than disciplinary purposes.

It is hoped these new arrangements will end the protracted delays, expensive suspensions on full pay and legalistic inflexibility of the old arrangements, although time will tell if this hope is realized in practice. National initiatives will only succeed if there is a change in the culture in which doctors work at a local level. The 'Three Wise Men' scheme has been shown to have serious weaknesses[15] and has been abolished.[16] Some Trusts are experimenting with alternative informal schemes to help deal at an early stage with conduct, health or performance issues. Offers of sabbatical leave may encourage doctors to reflect on their performance and develop their knowledge and skills. An environment is needed that promotes quality improvement, recognizes the inevitability of even good doctors making errors, and encourages openness and honesty about the performance of individuals and clinical teams. Such an environment, in which weaknesses can be identified and individuals can be helped to improve rather than be blamed, may offer the best chance for sustained quality improvement in healthcare.

Clinical governance and revalidation each have complementary advantages and disadvantages. Clinical governance can take swift action, proportional to the size of the problem, but cannot easily determine appropriate professional standards or easily prevent dangerous doctors from practising elsewhere. Revalidation, on the other hand, can provide a clear set of professional standards to support good practice and remove dangerous doctors from all forms of practice requiring registration, but cannot currently take very rapid action or easily deliver remedial solutions.

Since revalidation is a rolling process, with the revalidation decision being taken at five-yearly intervals, there should be plenty of opportunity for annual appraisal systems to identify gaps in the revalidation folders of individual doctors and for any action required to fill these gaps to be taken locally. There should therefore be no surprises at the end of the five-year period, since that small group of doctors who will not be recommended for revalidation are likely to have been identified well before this decision is made. Some doctors will have already been referred to the GMC under its fitness-to-practise arrangements, since if at any stage serious concerns are raised, they should be addressed immediately.

Quality assurance

As part of the GMC's quality assurance arrangements for revalidation, a random selection of doctors, including doctors to whom at least one predetermined key risk indicator applies, will be chosen in any submission year to submit their folders for greater scrutiny. Further details on sampling of folders is currently still awaited.

Healthcare services in the UK are subject to a variety of external review systems that, if working properly, should feed in to the revalidation process. Healthcare organizations have also increasingly used a variety of accreditation bodies to assess their level of performance in relation to established standards and to help implement ways of continuously improving the healthcare system. Many accreditation services focus on process and systems and not on performance of individuals; it is well recognized that good doctors can be struggling within dysfunctional teams, and vice versa. There is no reason, however, why the contribution of individuals to the overall performance of organizations should not be recognized in their revalidation folder.

Some specialist societies have developed peer review schemes and others are considering doing so. That organized by the British Thoracic Society was one of the first of such schemes and has been running since 1992.[17] A more recent one, based on the principles of *Good Medical Practice*, has been developed by the Association of Paediatric Anaesthetists.[18] Such schemes may, however, be more relevant to the development of local profiling processes than to the external review of them.

References

1. Irvine D. The performance of doctors. I: Professionalism and self regulation in a changing world. *BMJ* 1997; **314:** 1540–2.
2. *Good Medical Practice*, 3rd edn. London: General Medical Council, 2001.
3. *Continuing Professional Development*. London: General Medical Council, 2004.
4. Irvine D. The performance of doctors. II: Maintaining good practice, protecting patients from poor performance. *BMJ* 1997; **314:** 1613–15.
5. Smith J. The Shipman Inquiry. Dame Janet Smith (Chairman). Fifth Report. 2004: HMSO; 1027–1091.
6. *Good Practice. A Guide for Departments of Anaesthesia*, 2nd edn. London: Royal College of Anaesthetists and Association of Anaesthetists of Great Britain and Ireland, 2002.
7. Lack JA, White L, Thoms G, Rollin A-M. *Raising the Standard: A Compendium of Audit Recipes for Continuous Improvement in Anaesthesia*. London: The Royal College of Anaesthetists, 1999.
8. Godwin R, deLacey G, Manhire A. *Clinical Audit in Radiology: 100+ recipes*. London: The Royal College of Radiologists, 1996.
9. *Good Medical Practice for General Practitioners*. London: Royal College of General Practitioners and BMA GP Committee, 1999.
10. *A Guide to Standards in Private Practice*. Private Practice Forum, 1997. London: Academy of Royal Medical Colleges.
11. *The Future Organisation of Prison Healthcare*. London: HM Prison Service and NHS Executive, 1999.
12. *A First Class Service. Quality in the NHS*. London: Department of Health, 1998.
13. *Supporting Doctors, Protecting Patients*. London: Department of Health, 1999.
14. http://www.publications.parliament.uk/pa/pabills.htm.
15. Rosenthal MM. *The Incompetent Doctor: Behind Closed Doors*. Milton Keynes: Open University Press, 1995.
16. Maintaining High Professional Standards in the Modern NHS. Department of Health 2005. (available from www.dh.gov.uk)
17. Page RL, Harrrison BDW. Setting up interdepartmental peer review. The British Thoracic Society's scheme. *J R Coll Phys Lond* 1995; **29:** 319–24.
18. Crean PM, Stokes MA, Williamson C, Hatch DJ. Quality in paediatric anaesthesia: a pilot study of interdepartmental peer review. *Anaesthesia* 2003; **58:** 543–8.

12 Quality and clinical governance in out-of-hours care

Simon Mitchell

Introduction

The NHS is engaged in a process of systematically reviewing and improving all aspects of the care it provides. There have been many recent changes in the provision of out-of-hours care, and this chapter examines those changes from a quality perspective.

Background

The organization and structure of out-of-hours services have changed greatly during the course of this current parliament. The changes in structure and organization have principally been driven by the New General Medical Services contract that has given GPs the option to opt out of the responsibility for providing out-of-hours services. The responsibility for commissioning a service to provide out-of-hours care lies with the Primary Care Trusts (PCTs). PCTs across the country have taken different approaches to commissioning this service stream. All providers, however, have to be able to demonstrate that they meet the centrally set quality guidelines that were initially laid down in the Carson report.[1] These standards have been updated and are colloquially known as the 'New Carson Standards'; officially, these are *The National Requirements in The Delivery of Out-of-Hours Services*.[2]

The Report contains 13 quality standards, these are, in synopsis, as follows:

1. Providers must report regularly to PCTs on compliance with the standards.
2. Details of all out-of-hours contacts must reach a patient's registered practice by 08:00 the next day.
3. Providers must have mechanisms to allow regular exchange of up-to-date and comprehensive data between organizations.

4. There must be regular audits of contacts, and actions from those audits are to be carried out.
5. There must be regular audits of patient experience.
6. Providers must operate a complaints procedure in line with NHS procedure.
7. Providers must demonstrate an ability to match capacity to demand.
8. An initial telephone call is to be answered within 60 seconds (30 if there is no introductory message)
9. Clinical telephone assessment must identify all life-threatening conditions within 3 minutes, with definitive assessment to commence within 20 minutes for urgent calls and 60 minutes for non-urgent patients.
10. Face-to-face assessments should commence within 20 minutes of the patient arriving at the centre for urgent cases and 60 minutes for non-urgent patients. Life-threatening emergencies have to be identified within 3 minutes and be directed to the appropriate resource.
11. Providers must ensure that care is provided by the clinician best equipped to meet the patient's needs.
12. Face-to-face consultation must commence within 1 hour for emergencies, 2 hours for emergencies and 6 hours for all others, at the most appropriate location.
13. An interpretation service must be available within 15 minutes if required.

It is of course essential that all elements of the service meet the criteria also laid down in the recent publication *National Standards, Local Action.*[3]

Out-of-hours services

The new primary medical care contract (nGMS) has, for the first time, defined what constitutes normal working hours for primary care. These are 08:00 to 18:30 Monday to Friday, excluding bank holidays. All other hours are deemed to be 'out of hours'.

Primary Care Trusts have a responsibility to ensure that all their registered patient population can receive timely and appropriate medical care at all times. This care must be provided by an accredited provider. In some cases, the accredited provider may be the patient's own GP who has declined the opportunity to hand over the responsibility for providing out-of-hours cover to his own patients.

The PCT must ensure that providers of out-of-hours services meet the nationally agreed standards as laid down in the Carson Report. This can be done in a number of ways, for example monthly statistical reports and quarterly visits to providers. In monitoring such services, PCTs must be sure that the providers are not only complying with their contractual responsibilities but also meeting the national quality standards.[3]

PCTs must also be wary that if patients lose faith in the new services, this may have a knock-on effect in additional A&E attendances. This may have already happened in some areas, and Cardiff Local Health Board is actually evaluating the impact on local healthcare services.

Providing timely care

The document *National Quality Requirements in the Delivery of Out-of-Hours Services*[2] outlines what are considered to be appropriate response times to the request for medical help during the out-of-hours period. A summary reminder of these includes:

- initial telephone call – all calls answered within 60 seconds
- telephone or face-to-face clinical assessment – commence in urgent cases in 20 minutes, and in all others in 60 minutes
- face-to-face consultation – commences in urgent cases in 20 minutes, and in all others in 60 minutes

A monthly statistical report to the commissioning PCT outlining the achievement against these standards can be an adequate way of monitoring whether these targets are achieved.

Out-of-hours services must be able to cope with variable demand. It is particularly important for providers and PCTs to agree escalation policies to ensure that these standards are still met when there is high demand. Recently, a patient in Bristol complained that it took over 6 hours for a GP to attend to certify his wife's death. All around the country, there are numerous reports of these standards being breached.

Skill mix

After some initial prevarication, the Government has responded to patient concerns and stipulated that patients must be able to access a GP at all times if it is appropriate to do so. This has put some pressure on providers who felt that the time was ripe to move away from a GP-led out-of-hours service, and nationally the role of nurse practitioners in the delivery of out-of-hours care has been developed. However, most providers deliver high-quality care with a blend of traditional (GPs) and innovative staff. The role of nurses in triage is well established, and many providers are now extending the use of nurse practitioners into the team working to well-developed evidence-based protocols. One GP co-op has pioneered the use of physician assistants in out-of-hours care within the UK. Many other new roles are being developed to extend the team and embrace new roles for ambulance staff, district nurses, health visitors and psychiatric response teams.

Clearly, the use of extended teams facilitates the delivery of prompt care in response to patient demands and balances the requirement to have cost-effective packages of care with the need to ensure GP involvement. But the challenge for the providers and commissioners of out-of-hours services is to ensure that all clinicians involved are competent and fully trained and that staff are appropriately supervised.

A plethora of new roles have been developed and some have been embraced – for example, the medical press is littered with advertisements for jobs that are solely for GPs who wish to deliver out-of-hours care. Whatever role is created, those staff must have the right skills and competences to deliver care to a high standard. PCTs must therefore ensure that these individuals are included in educational programmes, appraisal and other clinical governance activities. Providers should endeavour to ensure that all clinicians have their work reviewed by their peers to ensure that clinical and record-keeping standards are maintained at an appropriate standard.

Patient involvement

In this age of the patient-centred NHS, it goes without saying that patients' views must be actively collected. Any new service, be it an orthopaedic service redesign or an out-of-hours service redesign, should be organized around patient require-ments and be developed in partnership with patients and the public. In this way, it is more likely that the new service will meet with approval from users. Com-munity groups, town teams, practice patient participation groups, etc. provide a number of fora that can be accessed and used to test new service models.

Clearly, patient and public involvement does not stop once a service is up and running; it is essential to seek out feedback from users to gauge their satisfaction and glean ideas for improvement. The need to get users' opinion is embedded in the new NHS primary care services contract and the wider NHS; indeed, the New Carson Standards stipulate that providers need to interview 1% of all users each quarter and develop an effective feedback mechanism on patient satisfaction. Perhaps more important is the need to reflect on the information generated by this approach and implement the changes required to improve the quality of the care delivered. The outcomes of those interviews should certainly be made available to the PCT commissioners.

An explicit complaints procedure need to be in place so that service users know where they can raise issues. Such a procedure needs to mirror those in the broader NHS and comply with national requirements. Any complaints that are received should be dealt with promptly and investigated appropriately, and the complainant should be kept informed of progress; the response should seek to reassure patients that appropriate action has been taken to improve service delivery and its quality. The details of and the response to the complaints should be forwarded to the PCT. The content of the complaints should be monitored and trend-analysed to make sure that areas needing improvement are identified. Out-of-hours clinical teams should receive this information at least quarterly so that they can identify which aspect of the service needs improvement.

Continuity of care

One of the most valuable aspects of the existing system of primary care within the UK is that it is built on a central pillar of continuity of care. This is highly valued by patients and also by the majority of practitioners. However, many changes are occurring to the way in which primary care is delivered during normal hours, which are eroding some of this continuity. The increasing use of IT systems within practices help shore up the impression the patient has of continuity in care.

Any out-of-hours service should endeavour to offer some semblance of continuity of care by the prompt and accurate transmission of clinical information back to individual practices. The contractual obligation stipulates that this information should be delivered by 08:00 the following day. This is of course a two-way process: practices must ensure that their patients are well informed regarding how to contact the out-of-hours provider and also that they give appropriate information to the out-of-hours provider about patients with particular problems (e.g. those who are terminally ill).

As these last two items are part of the Quality and Outcome Framework of the nGMS contract, PCTs therefore have the ability to monitor the passage of information both from and to practices. But it is important to remember that confidentiality has to be respected and that there is a need to have clear 'protocols' for sharing information.

Medicines management

PCTs throughout the UK have in general employed prescribing advisers whose role has been to encourage and develop quality-driven cost-effective prescribing. Central to this has been the development of mechanisms to feed back to practitioners on the quality of their own prescribing and that of their peers. This has often been coupled with educational programmes and incentive schemes that have resulted in better profiles of prescribing.

There are many aspects of prescribing in the out-of-hours services that have traditionally been a cause for concern, and many of these should be addressed by linking providers with appropriate advice from prescribing advisors.

Providers should now be linking their prescribing to the formulary of their commissioning PCT, and where possible receiving appropriate feedback from the prescribing advisers regarding compliance with the formulary.

PCT prescribing advisers should also be able to facilitate the procurement of medicines for use in the out-of-hours period rather than allowing pharmaceutical companies to be involved in supply.

A major concern over the years has been the limited availability of drugs for palliative care during the night. Prescribing advisers have been able to work with pharmacies and providers to ensure that this is no longer a cause for concern. This aspect of care, however, needs regular review.

There is a suggestion within the New Carson Standards that patients attending an out-of-hours provider for an episode of care should receive a full course of treatment there and then. Traditionally, patients have received enough tablets to see them through until a pharmacist can dispense a full course of medication, and often these interim tablets have been supplied without patient information leaflets, which is no longer acceptable. This is a high hurdle and one that many providers might struggle to meet without flexible thinking and support from the PCTs. The standard may yet be watered down, but the central theme of simple patient journeys will remain a yardstick within out-of-hours performance. Regular audits should be undertaken and the results shared with the PCTs.

Innovation in service delivery

In many parts of the country, there has been a move to integrate primary and secondary care out-of-hour services by co-locating primary care out-of-hours services with A&E departments. This has been done in part as a response to the Government's *Reforming Emergency Care*.[4] This publication highlights many problems with the existing tiers of service to patients who need unscheduled care. One recurrent theme is that patients often find themselves reciting their history to multiple professionals in several locations before finally receiving the care they need. By merging services and adopting a 'see and treat' approach, patients avoid the need to see a number of different staff members, and also get treated promptly by an appropriately trained professional in a single geographical location. There is a tremendous opportunity to involve GPs in this role, working at the front end of an emergency centre seeing both primary and secondary care attendees and linking appropriately with other services when necessary.

If this model of care is to develop further, it will be essential to ensure that all staff have been appropriately trained and have the skills competences required for the role. To ensure consistency in the way in which these roles are developed, A&E consultants and primary care providers will need to establish what core skills are required and develop a relevant training programme that will deliver highly skilled staff. Again, it will be necessary to monitor patient satisfaction with such services and have in place effective mechanisms to obtain their feedback and ensure that clinical teams have received this information to underpin their continuous improvement strategies.

Patient safety

Patients need to be reassured that they will not be harmed when coming into contact with out-of-hours services. As the configuration of such services is changing and being delivered by a range of staff with new roles, it is becoming increasingly important to ensure that appropriate systems are in place to identify potential risks and to capture untoward events, whether or not they result in harm. To this end, sound clinical risk management processes need to be introduced, with effective incident reporting. The information thus generated needs to be considered alongside other sources of clinical information by clinical teams in order to identify where changes in clinical and organizational practice need to occur.

Location and patient safety

The underlying theme of patient safety runs throughout the discussion of quality in out-of-hours services. It is essential that patients receive care from adequately trained professionals who act in an appropriate manner. It is of equal importance that the care be delivered in a safe environment. Commissioners must ensure that contracting arrangements ensure that buildings from which care is delivered are well maintained, fit for their purpose and compliant with all appropriate statutory legislation, especially the Disability Discrimination Act.

Services also need to be delivered from centres that are accessible to as many patients as is possible. Many services cover populations who have well below national average car ownership, and good public transport links are therefore essential. PCTs therefore need to take this issue into consideration when commissioning for out-of-hours services.

Lines of communication

Some aspects of communication that are required to ensure that patients receive quality care have already been dealt with. There are, however, several other issues that require consideration.

Many agencies are involved in the provision of unscheduled care. Processes should be developed to ensure that all professionals delivering aspects of this care are aware of the existence of other services and how to access them. I spent many hours one evening arranging for the section of a young boy with learning difficulties – a task made much more complicated by the lack of available information concerning roles and responsibilities of different crisis teams in social and psychiatric services.

PCTs should encourage providers to exchange information and link up services. This will be greatly facilitated once the technical hubs are set up to link providers with NHS Direct, but could be made a requirement of the contract with out-of-hours providers.

Intermediate care and quality

The shrinking number of secondary care beds and the need to admit patients from A&E has led to conflicting pressures within the system, and a number of intermediate care provisions have been established. Payment by results and practice-based commissioning will drive further changes that may result in an increasing number of intermediate care beds in the community. The likelihood is that out-of-hours medical cover for these beds will be provided by GPs and primary care teams. Commissioners will thus need to satisfy themselves that the care provided in these units is of an appropriate standard and mirrors the quality-driven service that we see elsewhere in the new NHS.

And finally...

Patients receiving care from the NHS deserve a service of the highest quality. The challenge to PCTs and providers is to develop systems to ensure that the quality is there, that services evolve and that patients are engaged in service development and evaluation.

Many observers believe that the ultimate ambition of the NHS should be to offer care that is of the highest quality and available 24 hours a day 7 days a week with no delineation between in-hours and out-of-hours services. Individuals involved in out-of-hours provision should begin the journey towards that goal by ensuring that existing and developing services are of the highest quality.

References

1. *Raising Standards for Patients. New Partnerships in Out of Hours Care*. London: Department of Health, October 2000.
2. *National Quality Requirements in the Delivery of Out-of-Hours Services*. London: Department of Health, October 2004.
3. *National Standards, Local Action. Health and Social Care Standards and Planning Framework*. London: Department of Health, July 2004.
4. *Reforming Emergency Care*. London: Department of Health, October 2001.

Chronic disease and the implications for clinical governance

Myriam Lugon and Carol Singleton

Introduction

Chronic diseases are responsible for significant morbidity and mortality worldwide and, according to the World Health Organization, account for 46% of the burden of disease.[1] It has been reported that about 17.5 million people in the UK are suffering from a chronic condition. Around 60% of adults report a chronic health problem. Over three-quarters of these have more than one disease and around one-quarter of these will have three or more problems.[2]

The number of people with chronic disease is set to double by 2030. People with long-term conditions form 80% of GP consultations. Management of these conditions is complex. Around 50% of people do not take their medication as prescribed.

Providing services for people with long-term diseases is putting increasing pressure on healthcare resources and at last the NHS is waking up to the need to develop new ways of delivering chronic care. Increasingly, chronic diseases feature in the development of healthcare policies and of new ways of working across healthcare sectors and across professional boundaries.

Various elements of clinical governance are essential in supporting effective care for people with chronic conditions. Staff and patients require tailored training and development programmes, evidence-based care and its assessment through audit is crucial in producing best outcomes for patients, and accurate and timely information systems underpin care provision.

The implications for clinical governance cannot be considered without examining the policy context and the organization and distribution of these services. These elements are discussed in this chapter.

Policy influences

The Department of Health has put the management of chronic diseases high on its agenda, and this culminated earlier this year in the publication, among others, of two national documents aiming to shape the way chronic care is delivered: *Supporting People with Long Term Conditions: an NHS and Social Care Model to Support Local Innovation*[2] and *The National Service Framework for Long Term Conditions*. While the latter deals primarily with long-term neurological conditions, the principles can be applied to other chronic diseases. The Department of Health has set targets for long-term conditions in *National Standards, Local Action*,[3] including:

> 'To improve health outcomes for people with long term conditions by offering a personalised care plan for vulnerable people most at risk; and reduce emergency bed days by 5% by 2008 (from the expected 2003/04 baseline), through improved care in primary care and community settings for people with long term conditions.'

In the USA, chronic disease management has been a priority of healthcare organizations for many years, and models of care based on a managed care approach have been developed. Such models include those from Kaiser Permanente, Evercare and the Legacy Health System,[4-7] for example. In most cases, the approach involves risk stratification within the population served, and targeting resources at high- and medium-risk individuals. For example, the Kaiser Permanente model includes level 2 (poorly controlled conditions needing care management) and level 3 (patients with multiple complex diagnosis needing case management). In all cases, information is an important element of good management, and all systems need to have suitable IT systems to support care.

The US approach to chronic disease management has led to significant service redesign and has also emphasized the importance of self-management. Research has shown that programmes teaching self-management are more effective than information alone and that, in the case of arthritis sufferers, self-management education can improve outcomes and reduce costs.[8] A 'major rethinking of primary practice' is necessary to manage chronic disease effectively within primary care.[9] Five essential elements for successful chronic care have been identified: support for self-management, decision support, clinical information, availability of community resources and how healthcare is organized.[9]

The UK has looked to the USA to develop its own approach. The Evercare model, based on identification of high-risk individuals, which has been piloted in nine Primary Care Trusts (PCTs), has been a catalyst for change and has led to hospital admission avoidance, decreased length of stay, improved quality of life and a more seamless approach to the delivery of care.[7] The NHS and Social Care Model[2] advocates case management for patients with complex and high-intensity needs, the use of protocols and care pathways for the management of specific diseases, and support for self-care. Community matrons[10] will deal with a caseload of up to 50 high-intensity patients. Their role includes organizing integrated care packages, preventing hospital admission whenever possible, and ensuring that patients are able to exercise choice; their work will take place within a primary care setting.

The approach to care within a health and social care economy

Both a population- and a patient-centred approach are prerequisites to ensuring access to appropriate care. The traditional model of care centred on specialist support from secondary care is rapidly becoming outdated. Increasingly, approaches to chronic care are centred on the patient's needs and are delivered within a community and primary care setting using primary care teams and a network of community providers[11] with support from specialists when necessary. This requires a change in the way in which services are designed. Importantly, a population-based approach also needs to be taken to ensure that services reach not only those in current receipt of support but all patients with chronic conditions who need to access care and to be seen and supported by healthcare professionals.[12]

The development of chronic care services needs to be underpinned by a number of principles agreed by all stakeholders. These principles should include the following:

- Enabling people to live as full a life as possible and to choose how their condition(s) should be managed.
- Empowering people to manage themselves.
- Offering support tailored to individual needs at home or in a community setting whenever possible.
- Making appropriate specialist support available when needed.
- Providing flexible care delivered by appropriately skilled staff.
- Ensuring that there is flexibility in the system to be able to respond to changing needs.

Socio-economic influences on chronic diseases are hugely important and must be considered when developing services for local populations. Addressing issues such as housing, transport, safety, security, financial support, isolation and community interaction is crucial in providing effective, holistic care. This approach requires close, effective interagency working across health, local authority services (e.g. housing, leisure, school and education), and the voluntary and private sectors.

There are a number of areas to address when developing a comprehensive model for the effective management of chronic disease within a community setting, many of which are described below.

A generic model of care emphasizing the importance of working with all sectors of the community to promote independence and provide effective support to patients with chronic conditions is shown in Figure 13.1. It highlights the need to empower people to take charge of their own condition, the need to work in partnership with various agencies in the public and voluntary sectors, and the requirement for effective communication and sharing of information, and it graphically demonstrates that the bulk of care is given outside traditional hospitals.

Maintaining health and well-being as well as preventing deterioration and the onset of a 'crisis' need to be emphasized as important elements of chronic disease management. Lifestyle education needs to feature in schools, but should also be made available to a range of different communities, including the population from ethnic minority groups that are prevalent in a health and

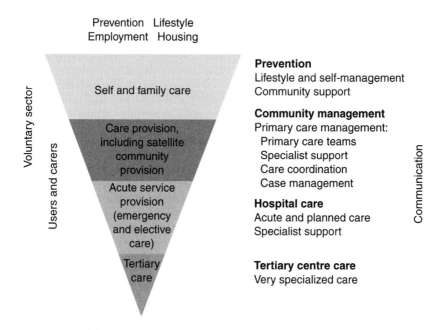

FIGURE 13.1 Model for chronic disease management.

social care economy. This will require equipping community staff (such as health visitors, school nurses, district nurses and community psychiatric nurses) with the skills needed to fulfil this important function.

It must be remembered that patients and their families will need time to come to terms with their disease as well as help to acquire the knowledge and skills to deal with their illness; in some cases, equipment for monitoring purposes will need to be provided.[2] The content of training and education programmes needs to be tailored to local needs, and the locations for delivery of the training (schools, the workplace, community centres, etc.) need to be appropriate for the local situation.

Patients with one or more diseases must be encouraged and supported to manage themselves, and programmes teaching self-management skills need to be developed and implemented. Within the UK, the Expert Patient programme has shown the benefits of patient education and empowerment, and it is being rolled out nationally.[13] There are huge opportunities for local health and social care economies to work with the voluntary sector in this area.

Patients should be diagnosed and initially be assessed in a primary care setting, where risk stratification is undertaken and a personalized care plan developed in partnership with each individual patient. The social context of the patient and their family and their need for information should influence how the care plan is constructed; the care plan should cover issues such as triggers for review, when care needs to be escalated, what to do in a crisis, and who to contact for advice and how. The care plan should be owned and held by the patient.

Patients with complex needs, identified as medium- and high-risk patients, require their care to be well coordinated, as it is likely to be provided by a number of different professionals; this coordination could be provided by appropriately skilled care coordinators with a finite case load – a role equivalent to that of community matrons.[10]

The way in which these patients could be managed is shown graphically in Figure 13.2.

Care coordinators will need to work in collaboration with members of individual primary care teams and hospital specialists, across the hospital and community interface, to ensure that care and support are given in the home whenever possible but in hospital where necessary. Part of their role needs to be to facilitate discharge of patients admitted for acute exacerbations of their condition as well as for some other reason, such as for elective surgery.

Specialist expertise should be made available outside existing hospitals and specialist clinics should be established within community settings, such as health centres; this will facilitate closer working relationship between hospital specialists and primary care physicians and improve communication.

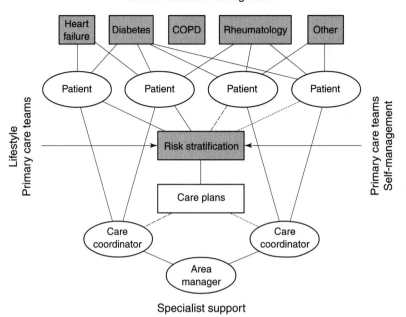

FIGURE 13.2 Management of patients with complex needs.

While the use of community matrons has been advocated to take the lead in management of patients in high-risk categories, this should not preclude the use of a range of healthcare workers to fulfil this role. For some patients, for example, it may be the hospital specialist nurse or consultant who best fits this role; for others, it may be a member of the primary health care team. Thus, within any health community, there will be a range of people coordinating care for patients with chronic conditions. The model proposes a management role to oversee this work so that cover for leave or sickness can be arranged when required.

Providing evidence-based care

Within the NHS, there is a history and culture whereby changes in clinical practice are more often the result of individual enthusiasm by clinical staff than a managed process.[14] Clinical aspects of the management of chronic conditions are often fairly well researched, but there is limited information on the organization of services.

Guidelines are well received where there are opportunities to tailor them to local needs.[15] The use of protocols ensures that care is evidence-based and consistent. 'Stepped care protocols' have been advocated as a means to manage chronically ill patients; by including explicit triggers based on clinical data,[12] the protocol can deal, for example, with issues such as when a referral to a specialist needs to be made. But systems for ensuring that protocols and guidelines are followed are often inadequate.

Proactive management of long-term conditions need to have explicit care pathways and protocols to ensure not only that the care delivered is evidence-based but also that there are effective strategies in place to reduce the need for hospital care and to improve outcomes, an approach advocated in the recently published document *Supporting People with Long-Term Conditions.*[2] While developed care pathways and protocols have usually been disease-specific, the needs of patients with more than one disease will need to be taken on board when developing local protocols; this in turn will inform what needs to be included in individual care plans. Pathways and protocols need to be locally developed/adapted with patient participation, locally owned, and regularly reviewed to remain in line with what is accepted as best practice; they should address not only how to deal with stable conditions but also what to do when there is an exacerbation. Further details on care pathways can be found in Chapter 4 of this book.

Clear monitoring strategies will also need to be in place to ensure that chronic conditions are effectively managed and that the service meets their needs; the strategy should cover *'whether to monitor at all, the choice of measurement(s), the choice of target range, the choice of measurement interval and who should monitor'*;[16] this should include self-monitoring.

Effective management of high-risk individuals requires prompt access to specialist support when needed (in a community setting whenever possible), easy access to diagnostics, and access to 'step-up' or 'step-down' facilities as appropriate for the needs of the patient. Local health and social care economies will need to consider how this is best provided in the light of available resources. For instance, 'rapid response' teams provide intensive short-term support in the community as an alternative to hospital admission and liaise with secondary care to shorten the length of stay of patients admitted to hospitals.

A number of areas across the country are experimenting with the use of technology in improving care for patients, including the use of assistive technology (such as Wristcare; North Lincolnshire PCT, personal communication) and structured telephone outreach programmes delivering disease-specific support.[17]

Efficient management of the patient in crisis is essential. One idea being considered and used in some health communities is provision of a single emergency number where calls are received by a call centre. If such an approach is taken, there must be '24/7' availability, 'response' protocols should be developed to ensure that patients are dealt with appropriately, calls should be logged, and any contact to the 'call centre' should trigger notification to the care coordinator and/or primary care team responsible for that patient.

Finally, consideration needs to be given on how to best measure the impact that this approach has on patients; here it is important to develop real outcome measures that are measures of the patient's experience and do not just concentrate on measuring the process. Examples of such outcome measures include the perceived intensity of symptoms such as pain, tiredness, depression and breathlessness.

What are the implications for clinical governance?

Effective delivery of chronic care needs a culture promoting a high quality of care and the use of improvement strategies[18] that are responsive to what chronic sufferers need and want. To this end, much more needs to be done to ensure that the views of these patients are sought and their feedback taken on board. The national Expert Patient programme goes some way towards empowering patients. But much more needs to be done at local levels to ensure that patients are involved in the clinical governance agenda and the development of services. Patients have a much broader perspective than individual healthcare professionals, as they come into contact with different parts of the healthcare system and understand what it means to live with a chronic condition; they can also inform what measure of outcomes will be of value to them and what would help them make informed decisions[19]. The views of users and carers can be sought in many ways, for example through interviews or focus groups, but some innovative approaches have also been used, such as giving patients disposable cameras to 'record their life' and to use these records to influence the views of healthcare professionals.[20]

The needs of people with long-term conditions are not always understood by healthcare professionals, and awareness of these must be raised.[21] This can be done by putting in place specific awareness training tailored to staff coming into contact with such individuals/patients and by ensuring that they have access to sources of information and support, for example, from the various local and national patient organizations and the Long Term Medical Alliance.

Audit plays an important role in monitoring clinical practice and service delivery. When pathways and protocols are developed, an audit tool needs to be created to allow prospective evaluation of the care delivered and the outcomes achieved, including quality-of-life measures as outlined above. Clinical teams and patients should be involved in determining how best to measure outcomes, so that the measures developed address what really matters to patients.

Audit should also be used to monitor and review the number of acute exacerbations suffered by patients with chronic disease, particularly when these seriously affect the ability of the patient to carry out the activities they wish and when they require admission to hospital. The audit should focus on the potential for avoidance of the problem in future, covering, for example, areas such as adequacy of regular care, medication prescribing and use, frequency of monitoring, and sufficient understanding from patient, carer and professional staff of the signs warning of deterioration. Healthcare organizations and their teams should also take part in national audits where such audits have been developed; these can act as an incentive for improvement and allow for comparators to be developed with similar institution.[22]

Measures of patient satisfaction with the care that they receive must also be included in a regular monitoring programme. The information generated in the process will help identify where changes are needed. As part of a robust audit process, time needs to be made available for teams to come together and review audit results together with all available clinical information (such as complaints and incidents), to reflect on current practice and to identify the next steps required.[23,24]

Agreement should be reached about the type of information (e.g. complaints, incidents, survey results, performance indicators, etc.) that is to be routinely collected, who is to collect it and who needs to receive it. This information should be regularly considered at team meetings alongside appropriate NICE guidelines, audit data and other relevant facts.

Health economy organizations will need to use their staff flexibly. A range of staff will need to acquire new skills and/or extend their role to support chronic disease management. This has major implication for the training and development agenda locally. The type of staff needed (e.g. professional and support staff) and the skills and competences that they require to manage and monitor people with long-term conditions must be dictated by the services that patients require. This may indicate that new roles are needed. Targeted training can then be developed and delivered. Some training areas are essential: these include the ability to assess risk and stratify patients accordingly and the ability to identify deterioration in a patient's condition as early as possible. The training programme should be formally accredited and appropriate career paths should be devised for staff moving into new roles.

The skills and competences of care coordinators and the training that they need require particular attention, as these staff will deal with the more complex patients – often those with more than one condition. The competencies required include understanding the chronic disease management process, knowledge of specific diseases and the ability to teach patients the skills to manage their own conditions (such as peak flow, blood pressure and sugar level monitoring). Care coordinators should also be able to work with groups, multidisciplinary teams and across organizational boundaries, have a degree of knowledge of what is available locally, and have good communication skills, but also need to be self-motivated, enthusiastic and willing to embrace changes. A range of staff, such as nurses, occupational therapists and physiotherapists, can fulfil this role, provided that they have, or can acquire, the necessary skills and competences to provide high standards of care.

Ongoing training and development will also need to be available. As care is delivered in teams, a 'team-based approach'[25] to learning should be considered. Training should also be provided across agencies and disciplines whenever possible. Other necessary training programmes include training and development for carers in residential and nursing homes to help to avoid unnecessary hospital admission.

Educating patients in how to manage their own disease and how to access relevant information is essential. Patients require advice and information about managing their medicines, the range of activities and support available from the statutory, private and voluntary sectors locally, who to contact when they want advice, where to find accessible information, and what to do if their condition flares up.

Staff working in different capacities and in different settings need to be clear about their roles, responsibilities and accountability. Effective supervision will ensure that staff work within the limits of their competences and that training needs can be identified. Healthcare organizations will need to agree who has overall responsibility for monitoring staff performance and provide access to relevant ongoing training and development.

Delivering chronic care is a complex endeavour; it involves many different staff from many different organizations; to avoid patients 'falling through the net', effective means of communication will need to be in place. Effective working will need to be underpinned by good IT systems in order to facilitate communication between the different sectors and the different professionals involved in the management of patients with chronic diseases. Because IT systems in the NHS are so fragmented, great attention needs to be paid to how healthcare systems can interface with each other and how health and social care systems can communicate with one another. Organizations will need to consider the type of information that they need to share, agree who has access to what, ensure timeliness and accuracy of information, agree principles for sharing information, and address confidentiality and security issues. Ideally, both patients and relevant staff should access care plans electronically. Robust information will need to be captured in appropriate databases not only to facilitate follow-up and monitoring of individual patients but also to make it easier for relevant staff to access the information that they need to care for those patients effectively.

Communication does not just concern healthcare professionals – communication with patients needs to be proactive: we can no longer assume 'that patients have relinquished control of their destiny to the clinicians'.[26]

Finally, to ensure that the care delivered is of a high standard, systems and processes such as the management of complaints, management of risk, audit, staff management and learning needs assessment will need to be robust and work across organizational boundaries. Primary care should take the lead responsibility to ensure that all necessary systems and processes are in place and are used by teams both as a learning tool and continuously to improve services.

Conclusion

The increasing burden of chronic disease requires a move from the traditional model of care delivery to a community- and primary care-focused approach with patients being empowered and supported to manage their condition(s) confidently themselves and supported by accessible, timely information. This requires close partnership working across statutory, private and voluntary agencies; it is necessary to be clear about respective roles and responsibilities not only of staff but also of their employing organizations. Clinical governance arrangements will need to transcend organizational boundaries, and the teams from different sectors will need to come together, with patients, to reflect and learn from what they do and to use continuous improvement strategies to ensure that patients with long-term conditions receive high-standard, evidence-based care.

References

1. WHO Global Strategy on Diet, Physical Acitivity and Health. Facts Related to Chronic Diseases: www.who.int/dietphysicalactivity/publications/facts/chronic/en.
2. *Supporting People with Long Term Conditions. An NHS and Social Care Model to Support Local Innovation*. London: Department of Health January 2005.
3. *National Standards, Local Action*. London: Department of Health, 2004.

4. Disease management in the American market. *BMJ* 2000; **320:** 562–6.
5. Griffith JR. Legacy Health System, Portland Oregon. In: *Designing 21st Century Healthcare.* 1998: Chapter 3. ACHE Management Series. Chapter 3. Health Administration PR 1998.
6. Kane R. Improving the management of chronic disease. *BMJ* 2003; **327:** 12.
7. *Implementing the Evercare Programme.* February 2004: www.natpact.nhs.uk.
8. Bodenheimer T *et al.* Patient self management of chronic disease in primary care. *JAMA* 2002; **288:** 2469–75.
9. Bodenheimer T *et al.* Improving primary care for patients with chronic illness. *JAMA* 2002; **288:** 1775–9.
10. *Supporting People with Long Term Conditions. Liberating the Talents of Nurses Who Care for Long Term Conditions.* 2005. The National Service Framework for Long Term Conditions. DOH 2005.
11. Wilson T *et al.* Rising to the challenge: Will the NHS support people with long term conditions? *BMJ* 2005; **330:** 657–61.
12. Gask L. Role of specialists in common chronic diseases. *BMJ* 2005; **330:** 651–3.
13. *The NHS Improvement Plan: Putting People at the Heart of Public Services.* London: Department of Health, June 2004.
14. *The Implementation of Clinical Effectiveness.* London: Clinical Standards Advisory Group, 1998.
15. Dunning M *et al. Experience, Evidence and Everyday Practice. Creating Systems for Delivering Effective Healthcare.* Kings Fund, 1999.
16. Glasziou P *et al.* Monitoring in chronic disease: a rational approach. *BMJ* 2005; **330:** 644–8.
17. Blackwater Valley and Hart PCT. *Health Serv J* 2005; 12 May: 31.
18. Lewis R *et al.* Rethinking management of chronic diseases. *BMJ* 2004; **328:** 220–2.
19. Kelson M. Patient involvement in clinical governance. In: *Advancing Clinical Governance,* Chapter 2. RSM Press 2001.
20. Fraser S, Wilson T, Burch K. Pictures really are worth a thousand numbers. *Clin Governance Bull* 2001; **2:** 15.
21. Levenson R, Joule N. *Improving People's Lives. The Agenda for People With Long Term Medical Conditions.* London: Long Term Medical Alliance, 1999.
22. Lugon M. Clinical audit. *Clin Governance Bull* 2005; **1:** 1–2.
23. Lugon M *et al.* Clinical audit. *Clin Governance Bull* 2002; **3:** 1–2.
24. Hewer P. Top tips for clinical audit. *Clin Governance Bull* 2002; **3:** 12.
25. Team based learning. In: Wakley G, Chambers R (eds). *Chronic Disease Management in Primary Care.* Oxford: Radcliffe, 2005.
26. Lugon M, Scally S. Communication. *Clin Governance Bull* 2001; **2(3):** 1–2.

Index